Nursing Homes to Rehabilitation Centers

Nursing Homes to Rehabilitation Centers

WHAT EVERY PERSON
NEEDS TO KNOW

• • •

Phyllis Ayman

Cover design by:
Natalie Bonilla, Graphic Designer
Minuteman Press, Stamford, CT
graphicsdesk@minutemanpress.com

Chandelier courtesy of:
Kristals Cosmetics
Greenwich, CT

ISBN: 1974131696
ISBN 13: 9781974131693
Library of Congress Control Number: 2017912076
CreateSpace Independent Publishing Platform
North Charleston, South Carolina

*This book is dedicated to all the patients and residents
in the skilled-nursing facilities and rehabilitation centers
with whom I have worked and from whom I have learned
so much, both personally and professionally.*

*A special thanks to Charlene Harrington, a staunch advocate of
improved care for the disabled, our elder citizens, and nursing home
quality care, who I called at the initial stages of this endeavor. She
was not only encouraging and supportive of my effort, but pointed
me in the direction of the all-important advocacy organizations:
Consumer Voice and the Long-Term Care Community Coalition.*

*I also want to thank my very dear friend and teacher, Suzanne
Swope, for her never-ending support, guidance, and input.*

*Last, but not least, many thanks to my daughter, Sarette, who
helped me prepare the manuscript for editing—I couldn't have
done it without you—and to my son, Graham, with whom I
have been able to share insights about personal growth.*

Contents

Prologue

• • •

My journey in nursing homes and rehabilitation centers is both personal and professional.

I remember my first visit to what was then Ingersoll Nursing Home, located a few blocks from my home. I was fifteen. I walked in the front door of the facility, and there was my grandmother seated in the lobby, slumped over in a wheelchair, unattended, and with a copious amount of saliva drooling out of her mouth onto her clothes—my kind, extremely proud, and pristine grandmother. The smell was nauseating. I was horrified.

Almost immediately after stepping foot inside the nursing-home door, I ran out. With the stench of urine in my nose, I walked around the block several times, tears streaming down my cheeks, before I could compose myself sufficiently to walk back inside to take care of Grandma. This was my first nursing-home experience, and it left an indelible mark on my mind and heart.

The decision to place my grandmother in the nursing home was an agonizing one. My grandmother's deteriorating condition was the result of Parkinson's disease and a broken hip. We lived in Brooklyn, New York, and she lived in the Bronx. My mother didn't drive, and I remember her making the one-and-a-half- to two-hour journey by bus and train to visit and care for my grandmother several times a week—leaving early in the morning and often returning after the family had eaten dinner.

After a considerable period of time, the routine began to take its toll on our family. Grandma's continued failing health made it clear that this schedule was not feasible on a long-term basis. My mother, being the eldest of three, wanted her to come live with us. My father, however—who was completely supportive of my mother's care for my grandmother—felt that her coming to live with us would be a strain. The hospital bed that she required would have taken up most of the living room, and he did not think that would be a good idea since I was a teenager who had friends over to the house on a regular basis. Furthermore, he felt that the entire family would be on constant call.

That is how the decision to place Grandma in the nursing home came to pass.

Shortly thereafter, when I was a junior in high school and just fifteen years old, my parents took a European trip to celebrate their twenty-fifth wedding anniversary. My sister, who was a twenty-two-year-old college student at Brooklyn College, had classes in the afternoon, and she and I agreed to take care of Grandma in their absence.

Every day my sister would visit Grandma, taking a nutritious eggnog drink my mother used to take for her, along with whatever clean clothes were washed from the night before. My sister would stay until early afternoon, when she had to leave for her classes, and I would go after school and stay through the dinner meal to feed her.

This was the impetus that framed my professional life.

After finishing high school, I went on to major in communication disorders at Emerson College in Boston, Massachusetts, where I completed my master of science degree in speech pathology at the University of Wisconsin–Madison. I was fortunate to land a well-paying, full-time job in Milwaukee right out of college—interestingly enough in a nursing home. My patients were primarily my current age or even older, and they were placed there because of lack of family or resources to care for them. Patients included those who had strokes, Parkinson's disease, dementia, and a myriad of other ailments often associated with older people.

I moved back to New York in 1977. My first job as a speech-language pathologist was at the prestigious Rusk Institute at NYU Medical Center. Later, after marriage and a baby, I moved to Westchester and took a break from nursing homes, concentrating on working in special education schools, special education preschools, hospitals, and private practice.

The nursing-home environment that had such a profound effect on me as a teenager continued to call to me. My first foray back into that setting was in a facility owned by a couple who had immigrated to the United States from Poland. That facility was soon bought out by a family who owned several facilities in the area; this was my first glimpse into the corporate world of nursing-home ownership. Over the next twenty-plus years, I have worked in forty nursing homes or rehabilitation centers; a few were not for profit, but most of them were for profit.

I've seen a lot—both favorable and unfavorable. Nursing homes have evolved over the years from places where we essentially warehouse our elderly citizens as we wait for them to die to skilled nursing facilities and rehabilitation centers. These centers are owned and operated, in many cases, by large corporations that thrive on gaming the system that funds patient care to increase profits and acquire more facilities. In many cases the nursing-home industry has become a perverse culture of doing the minimum for those in its care in order to maximize profits.

Most people have the impression that the system is entirely broken, but I postulate that the system is set up with the wrong reinforcers. It is reimbursement driven rather than patient- or quality-care driven. Thus, the manipulation and use of the system for material gain is the real culprit. Most of these owners have made, and continue to make, large profits off the elderly and infirm, draining every dollar—every penny—that they can to buy more facilities and make more money.

This fact became the impetus for this book: to focus attention on the gestalt—the problem as a whole—by revealing the truths and providing information about how the system functions from the inside.

I feel strongly that as we are in fact consumers of health care, and as such, we should be armed with the information as to how the nursing-home system operates. Once over the age of twenty-one, anyone who has a serious accident or illness may find himself or herself in a hospital, only to be discharged within a short time period. In the event the patient's home environment is not conducive to continued care or rehabilitation needs, he or she may inevitably wind up in a nursing home/rehabilitation center. Furthermore, as baby boomers are discovering, they are often confronted with decisions about the care of parents and older loved ones.

The national conversation on health care usually includes insurance for medical bills, hospitalization, preexisting conditions, pharmaceuticals and pharmacy companies, and more. Rarely, if ever, is there a mention of nursing homes or rehabilitation centers. There have been many issues related to health care that were once not part of the national conversation: Alzheimer's disease, breast cancer, mental-health issues, depression, and AIDs. It took strong voices and committed advocates who continued to openly discuss and consistently speak out on these issues until they ultimately became part of the conversation. Today there are people wearing ribbons for cancer, and there is a breast-cancer awareness month —as well as fashion events sporting the color red—dedicated to the all-important issue of heart disease among women. There are people wearing ribbons to support AIDS research for those members of the community affected by that dreadful disease.

National Nursing Home Awareness Week begins each year on Mother's Day, but I don't know of many people outside of the industry—or affiliated with it through family or friends—have any idea about its existence. In 1967 the American Health Care Association (AHCA) established the week to "provide an opportunity for residents and their loved ones, staff, volunteers, and surrounding communities to recognize the role of skilled nursing facilities in caring for America's seniors and individuals with disabilities."[1] As I read this, the question I had—and I believe every person should have—is "What about the care?"

The closest I came to any awareness of the event in the public domain was a tweet by a major TV personality in response to a May 2017 video production that extolled the thrill of being a staff member working at a particular facility. I have personal knowledge of that facility, and I can safely say that, while the video may have been a successful marketing tool to attract potential staff members, it did not accurately depict the functional environment of that particular nursing home/rehabilitation center.

In 2011, the Consumer Voice (National Consumer Voice for Quality Long-Term Care) expanded the period of time to focus on nursing home residents by establishing October as National Residents' Rights Month. It was established to highlight the lives of those who live in long-term care facilities and to focus awareness on the dignity, respect and rights to which they are entitled. Celebrating residents' rights began in 1981 as a way of paying tribute to residents. With the passage of the Nursing Home Reform Law of 1987, a week was established to honor nursing home residents. I have worked in 40 skilled nursing facilities/rehabilitation centers and haven't seen this celebrated or acknowledged with much significance, if at all.

The stories included in this book are firsthand accounts of my personal experiences or the experiences of my colleagues. I

---

1 "The Spirit of America," American Health Care Association, accessed July 2017, https://www.ahcancal.org/events/national_nursing_home_week/.

chose them to reflect the problematic issues related to nursing homes and rehabilitation centers. They are examples of how the policies, procedures, and laws are misapplied, negatively impacting the quality of care delivered to patients and residents. The stories are set apart from the chapter information by their descriptive titles and *distinctive print.*

It is my fervent hope that this book will increase awareness and raise the conversation about the nature of, and motivations for, the care provided in nursing homes and rehabilitation centers to a national level. We need to do better for our elder citizens and show them the respect they deserve for the years they have spent contributing to this country through their hard work. Knowledge can be a powerful tool and can help us to be strong advocates for ourselves and for our loved ones.

CHAPTER 1

From Nursing Homes to Rehabilitation Centers: How Did We Get Here?

• • •

THE MODERN-DAY USE OF THE words "nursing home" or "skilled-nursing facility" is a misnomer of sorts. (See appendix for a description of the difference between nursing homes [NH] and skilled nursing facilities [SNF].)

As we know them today, these facilities actually represent caregiving that is delivered on three different levels: (1) individuals who are acutely ill and require long-term custodial care (The facility becomes their home, thus the term "nursing home," and they are referred to as "residents."), (2) patients placed for transitional care, and (3) patients who are there for short-term rehabilitation.

The story of how the facilities themselves evolved dates back to the formation of our nation, and—as with many other social issues in our society—the history of how our nation has managed the care of our elders and infirm has been unsavory at best. This poor record is no more evident than in establishments that were known as almshouses, which were supported by landowner taxes and provided food and shelter.

Almshouses, which were based on an English concept, were first introduced into the Americas by William Penn, the founder of the Commonwealth of Pennsylvania. Though the notion of almshouses was originally charitable, providing food and shelter to older people who did not have the means or family to help care for them and who could no longer work, these places most often targeted the indigent, handicapped, elderly, or widows of the poorer segment of the community. One description depicts the utter dread of the situation. The elderly in these institutions oftentimes had to reside "alongside those that were insane, inebriated, or homeless,"[2] regardless of age. These plac-es came to be known as "poorhouses"—though being placed there was not necessarily associated with the person's financial situation—and along with that term came an incredible stigma.

With the arrival of the Industrial Revolution, more people moved to, or congregated near, urban areas for work, resulting in families dispersed throughout the county. This often left the aging without family support.

From this circumstance churches and women's groups es-tablished the first houses for the elderly; many of these were geared solely toward widows and single women with limited means. Some of the first homes were the Indigent Widows Single Women's Society in Philadelphia (1823) and the Home for the Aged Women in Boston (1850). But these homes were not open to all in need. There were considerable entrance fees, and in some instances references attesting to the woman's good character were required. Many of those in dire need were still relegated to almshouses.

One could say these homes perpetuated a kind of elitism that reinforced the social inequality and injustices of the times. The founders' concern was that "worthy individuals of their own ethnic or religious background might end their days along-side the most despised."[3] The statement made by the founder

---

2 *Encyclopedia of Aging Online*, s.v. "Nursing Homes: History," accessed August 2016, http://www.encyclopedia.com/education/encyclopedias-almanacs-transcripts-and-maps/nursing-homes-history.
3 C. Haber and B. Gratton, *Old Age and the Search for Security: An American Social History* (Bloomington: Indiana University Press, 1994), 130 (hereafter cited as *Old Age and the Search for Security*).

of the Boston's Home for Aged Women elucidates this point. The facility was "a haven for those who were bone of our bone and flesh of our flesh…and who expressed disdain for foreigners who…have taken possession of the public charities…as they have of the houses where our less privileged classes formerly resided."[4] There was a stark contrast between these institutions—benevolence and charitable care associated with church groups and women versus deplorable conditions associated with the almshouses.

Almshouses were the primary residences that cared for the elderly throughout the nineteenth century. There were also states that had "outdoor relief," where meager provisions of money, clothes, or wood were supplied as a means for survival so that the person could continue to live independently. However, this relief would intermittently be revoked, forcing the individual into the almshouse.

As the years went on, there was a shift in the diversity of the almshouse population due in large part to the organization of other institutional-type settings targeting younger people or dedicated to specific needs (e.g., orphanages, work homes, hospitals, or insane asylums). According to statistics, in 1880 33 percent of the population in the almshouses was comprised of the elderly; by 1923 that percentage had risen to 67 percent. The term "almshouse" seemed to lose its distinction as an appropriate name for these institutions, and in 1903 the Charity Board of the City of New York changed the name of its almshouse to

---

4 *Old Age and the Search for Security*, 130.

the Home for the Aged and Infirmed. Similarly, Charleston changed the name of its almshouse to the Charleston Home in 1913. The premise was that the elderly would be cared for and kept comfortable as they approached their final days within these homes.

By the early part of the twentieth century, there was an increase in social consciousness regarding the almshouses. The stigma of the almshouse as a poorhouse continued as Harry C. Evans, a noted social analyst of the time, described the environment: "a world of hate and loathing, for it includes the composite horrors of poverty, disgrace, loneliness, humiliation, abandonment, and degradation."[5] It became obvious that as the aged—as they were often referred to—could no longer work or care for themselves, they also became increasingly dependent upon the system. In 1929 Abraham Epstein, who was a well-respected advocate of pensions for the old, wrote that the almshouse "stands as a threatening symbol of the deepest humiliation and degradation before all wage earners after the prime of life."[6] However, despite the unsavory conditions for the elderly, who were relegated to enduring placement alongside those members of society who were mentally ill, homeless, or drug or alcohol dependent, almshouses became costly to operate. With the realization that a significant portion of the population would become increasingly dependent, there were those who felt that small pensions would be a suitable alternative.

---

5 A. Epstein, *The Challenge of the Aged* (New York: Alfred A. Knopf, 1929), 218 (hereafter cited as *The Challenge of the Aged*).

6 *The Challenge of the Aged*, 128.

The Social Security Act of 1935 considered pensions in light of the increasing elderly population in the almshouses. Those who advocated pensions for people no longer able to work also felt strongly that those within the almshouses should not be able to receive any income. The thought process was that if the elderly were given financial means they would be able to care for themselves and thus eliminate the need for the almshouse. This would finally eradicate from society the degradation and humiliation associated with those institutions. Conversely those who lived in privately funded institutions would be allowed to receive pensions. The matter went all the way to the Supreme Court, whereby Supreme Court Justice Benjamin Cardozo, a renowned legal scholar of the times, wrote in his majority opinion, "The hope behind this statute is to save men and women from the rigors of the poorhouse as well as the haunting fear that such a lot awaits them when the journey's end is near."[7]

It became increasingly obvious that though a small percentage of those residing in the almshouses were there due to dire financial circumstances, the larger percentage consisted of the elderly, frail, physically ill, or infirm who were unable to care for themselves or who were beyond the reaches of other in-home care—even with the allocation of pension funds.[8]

This vacuum created by eliminating the almshouse gave rise to a dilemma of different proportions. Those receiving pension

---

7 R. L Tullis, *Benjamin Nathan Cardoza: Jurist, Philosopher, Humanitarian* Louisiana Law Review (1938) Volume 1/Number1 accessed September 2017 http://digitalcommons.law.lsu.edu/lalrev/vol1/iss1/19, 151

8 W. C. Thomas, *Nursing Homes and Public Policy* (Ithaca, NY: Cornell University Press, 1969), 40.

payments who were in continued need of long-term care had to seek alternative places to reside in their final days. Many entered privately owned institutions that were unregulated. In many cases these were the same almshouse-type institutions with the names changed but consisting of the same players. The residents of these institutions were now under the auspices of a private-care system, thereby allowing the inhabitants' monthly pensions to be diverted to the institution.

By the 1950s both the almshouses and poorhouses were essentially eradicated. Social Security had been successfully amended, and residents in public facilities were now able to receive federal funding. In 1954 the passage of the Medical Facilities Survey and Construction Act allowed those residing in both public and private facilities to receive federal assistance, affirming the realization that a substantial number of the elderly could not sustain themselves outside of an institution despite receiving pension funds.

Medicare and Medicaid were two of the most important programs created as a result of the Social Security Amendments of 1965, the purpose of which was to create federal health insurance for those over the age of sixty-five (at that time referred to as the elderly), as well as for poor families. These programs helped facilitate the rapid growth of the nursing-home industry. One statistic indicates that from 1960 to 1976 there was a 140 percent increase in the number of nursing homes nationally, with a concomitant rise in revenue of 2,000 percent. The proliferation of these facilities was primarily related to the entrance of private ownership into this arena. By 1976 79 percent of the nation's elderly who resided in these facilities did so in those that were owned or operated by private industry.

However, the rise of the nursing-home industry did not solve the issue of care for our aging population. The reputation of these facilities was little better than the almshouses, replete with stories of poor or substandard care and insufficient medical care, food, and staffing and were characterized by a rather gruesome description of being little more than a warehouse or junkyard for those that were old or dying. There were cries for reform, and nursing homes were described as "halfway houses between society and the cemetery."[9] As with the almshouse, there was a growing fear on the part of individuals and their family members—who had to face the feelings that they were abandoning their loved ones—that one would wind up essentially waiting to die in one of these facilities.

In 1971 the outcry finally led to increased government regulation to oversee the quality of long-term care through the Office of Nursing Home Affairs. This office was responsible for oversight, and it established standards of practice. Along with those reforms, there was also reform that applied to facilities receiving Medicare and Medicaid dollars. In addition, there was other legislation—notably the Older Americans Act of 1973 and the Federal Nursing Home Reform Act of 1987, which was included in the passage of the Omnibus Budget Reconciliation Act (also called OBRA '87)—that President Ronald Reagan signed into law.

---

9 R. N. Butler, *Why Survive: Being Old in America* (New York: Harper and Row, 1975), 263.

The Federal Nursing Home Reform Act of 1987 is widely considered the first major revision of the federal standards and practices for nursing-home care since 1965, when both Medicare and Medicaid were created. The legislation effectively changed the landscape for legal ramifications and expectations for individuals residing in nursing homes, and it specifically stated, "long-term care facilities wanting Medicare or Medicaid funding are to provide services so that each resident can attain and maintain his/her highest practicable physical, mental, and psychosocial well-being."[10] It also created an ombudsman program that was essentially a means for residents and families to voice complaints about any infringement of their care or their overall well-being to an impartial proprietor of sorts who would advocate on their behalf.[11]

The changes that OBRA '87 outlined as essential for nursing-home care are as follows:

- Emphasis on a resident's quality of life as well as quality of care
- New expectations that each resident's ability to walk, bathe, and perform other activities of daily living (ADLs) will be maintained or improved with obvious consideration given to medical reasons
- A resident-assessment process leading to development of an individualized care plan

---

10 M. Klauber and B. Wright, "The 1987 Nursing Home Reform Act," AARP, accessed September 2016, http://www.aarp.org/home-garden/livable-communities/info 2001/ the_1987_nursing_home_reform_act.html

11 R. C. Atchley, *Social Forces and Aging* (Belmont, CA: Wadsworth Publishing, 1994), 511.

- Rights to remain in the nursing home absent nonpayment, dangerous resident behaviors, or significant changes in medical condition
- New opportunities for potential and current residents with mental retardation or mental illnesses for services inside and outside of the nursing home
- A right to safely maintain or bank personal funds with the nursing home
- Rights to return to the nursing home after a hospital stay or an overnight visit with family and friends
- The right to choose a personal physician and to access medical records
- The right to organize and participate in a resident or family council
- The right to be free of unnecessary and inappropriate physical and chemical restraints
- Uniform certification standards for Medicare and Medicaid homes
- Prohibition on turning to family members to pay for Medicare and Medicaid services
- New remedies to be applied to certified nursing homes that fail to meet minimum federal standards

Despite the landmark reform, the standards for care in all nursing homes did not change significantly, and to this day many people continue to fear placement in a skilled nursing or nursing-home facility. What is noteworthy is that as a society our life expectancy has increased, so the average age of the nursing-home resident has steadily increased to present-day numbers. Whereas in 1990 only 1 percent of the population in nursing homes was between sixty-five and seventy-four years old, that number was 25 percent for the eighty-five-plus population.[12] That number continues to grow, and today individuals eighty-five years and older, sometimes described as the "oldest old" and colloquially known as the "graying of America," are considered to be the portion of the population seeing the most rapid growth. In 2012 the estimated number of individuals eighty-five years and older in the United States was 5.9 million.[13] This figure is expected to increase to 19.4 million by 2050.[14]

However, not all persons in need of long-term care are elderly. Approximately 63 percent are persons aged sixty-five and older (6.3 million); the remaining 37 percent are sixty-four years of age and younger (3.7 million).[15] Today it is estimated that a senior citizen of age sixty-five or older has about a one-in-four chance of spending some time in a nursing home or skilled-nursing facility. As families become more dispersed, there is a stark possibility of placement in one of these facilities that many older adults do not want to face—nor do their families.

---

12 *"Sixty-Five Plus in the United States"* Statistical Brief: U.S. Census Bureau May 1995 accessed September 2017 https://www.census.gov/population/socdemo/statbriefs/agebrief.html

13 "A Profile of Older Americas: 2013," Administration for Community Living, accessed September 2017, https://www.acl.gov/sites/default/files/Aging%20and%20Disability%20in%20America/2013_Profile

14 "U S Census Bureau Statistical Abstract of the United States: 2000," US Census Bureau, accessed September 2017, http://www.census.gov/prod/2004pubs/.

15 S. Rogers and H. Komisar, *Who Needs Long-Term Care? Fact Sheet, Long-Term Care Financing Project* (Washington, DC: Georgetown University Press, 2003), http://www.aaltci.org/long-term-care-insurance/learning-center/long-term-care-statistics.php.

The landscape of the typical nursing-home environment has also changed dramatically. As hospitals discharge patients sooner, striving to cut costs in light of reduced insurance reimbursement for extended stays, many people are in need of transitional services to address continuing medical and rehabilitation needs. Thus, most of these facilities have active, short-term rehabilitation units, also known as "subacute," which often involve Medicare dollars and where high reimbursement for a one-hundred-day stay allows patients to be rehabilitated sufficiently to return to their prior living situation. However, it should also be noted that anyone over the age of twenty-one in need of intensive therapy services can be placed in a subacute unit in one of these facilities.

The emphasis on short-term Medicare has become more desirable due to the reimbursement rate, which is approximately 84 percent higher than the facility would otherwise receive from Medicaid or private health insurance. This has resulted in a trend where some facilities and companies are eliminating all long-term-care and Medicaid beds in favor of the higher, short-term Medicare reimbursements. According to a federal data report, the percentage of residents covered by Medicare in nursing homes rose from 9 percent in 2000 to 15 percent in 2014.[16]

The Congressional Budget Office (CBO) reported figures with more specificity. It estimated that expenditures on long-term care totaled more than $120 billion in 2000, calculating

---

16 "2014 CMS Statistics," US Department of Health and Human Services, accessed September 2017, https://www.cms.gov/Research-Statistics-Data-and-Systems/Statistics-Trends-and-Reports/CMS-Statistics-Reference-Booklet/Downloads/CMS_Stats_2014_final.pdf.

that 59 percent of all the expenses were covered by the public sector (Medicare and Medicaid). The balance was largely covered by out-of-pocket expenses accounts, while private insurance covered just 1 percent of the long-term-care costs (see graph that follows). Conservative CBO estimates suggest that total long-term-care expenditures will increase at a rate of 2.6 percent per year above inflation over the next thirty years, shooting to $154 billion in 2010, $195 billion in 2020, and a whopping $270 billion in 2030. These numbers do not account for changes in the use of long-term-care insurance, which may become more common. If is the case, the dramatic upward trend in long-term-care reimbursement expenditures will continue.[17]

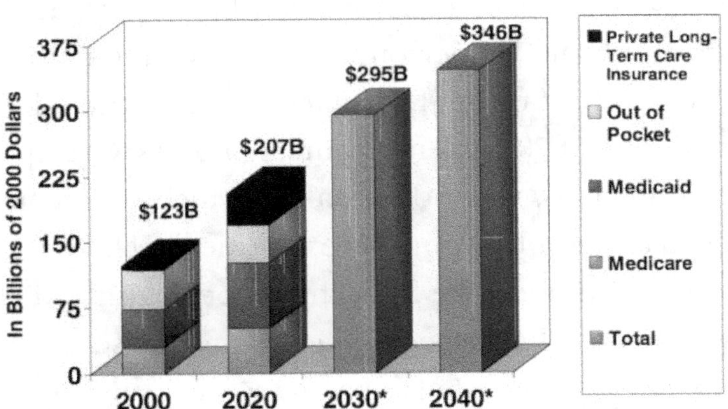

Source: "Projections of expenditures for long-term care services for the elderly," CBO 1999
Dollar totals in 2030 and 2040 are not disaggregated by payer due to uncertainty about projections. [18]

---

17 S. Corbin-Jallow and R. Moore, "CBO Memorandum: Projections of Expenditures for Long-Term Care Services for the Elderly," Congressional Budget Office, http://www.dtic.mil/get-tr-doc/pdf?AD=ADA399651.

18 J. R. Knickman and E. K. Snell, "The 2030 Problem: Caring for Aging Baby Boomers," Health Services Research, accessed September 2017, https://www.ncbi.nlm.nih.gov/pmc/articles/PMC1464018/#b13.

This has created a rather undesirable, albeit pernicious, situation where individuals—or more commonly corporations—assemble groups of investors to acquire more buildings, seizing on the opportunity to create long-term-care or rehabilitation centers. They compete with one another to woo patients with luxury lobbies and amenities, state-of-the-art rehabilitation departments, redesigned rooms, specialized menu preferences, and an emphasis on quality, individualized service.

The Centers for Medicare & Medicaid Services (CMS) began collecting information on nursing-home ownership in 2003 via homes that received reimbursement as a participating provider in the Medicare program. It found the information, which was largely self-reported, somewhat convoluted and difficult to unravel for both the lay person as well as for regulatory agencies.[19] A 2008 report by the Department of Health and Human Services found that 70 percent of nursing homes were operating on a for-profit basis, more than half of which were controlled by chains made up of two or more facilities.[20] There was actually an instance whereby the Department of Health and Human Services' Office of the Inspector General found seventeen limited liability companies listed as having some involvement in the ownership for one nursing-home facility being investigated for substandard care.[21]

---

19 *Nursing Home Enforcement: Collection of Civil Monetary Penalties*, Office of Inspector General, accessed August 2017, https://www.oig.hhs.gov/oei/reports/oei-06-03-00420.pdf.
20 *2008 Agency Financial Report*, Section III-23 Health and Human Services, 11/17/2008; Updated 12/08/2008 accessed March 2017, https://www.hhs.gov/about/agencies/asfr/finance/financial-policy-library/agency-financial-reports/index.html See Archive of HHS Financial and Performance Reports (hereafter cited as *2008 Agency Financial Report*).
21 *2008 Agency Financial Report*.

In addition, each facility strives to find its own market niche to attract the highest-paying customers (i.e., orthopedic [hips, knees, shoulder repairs] or cardiac rehabilitation and other specialties). The term that has been coined to describe this trend is the "chandelier effect." Many of these units face the same challenges noted in other parts of the facility: understaffed and poorly trained nursing assistants and nurses and limited visits by a medical doctor in favor of a nurse practitioner (NP) or physician's assistant (PA).[22]

Furthermore, some of the worst offenders, in an attempt to lure Medicare patients, market amenities and high-quality care and rehabilitation when that is not what they deliver. A *New York Times* article described such a situation at a Long Island facility that opened a short-term rehabilitation wing where patients (called "guests") had access to a putting green, model apartment, and a parked PT Cruiser to teach them how to resume their day-to-day activities. Despite these amenities the New York attorney general sued the facility for circumstances related to quality care that resulted in a death of a patient. The facility was ultimately placed on a federal watch list for being among the nation's poorest-performing facilities.[23]

---

22 "Nursing Homes Compete with Lavish Amenities for Short-Term Rehabilitation Residents," August 2015 Gallivan and Gallivan New York Nursing Home Abuse Lawyer Blog, accessed March 2017, https://www.newyorknursinghomeabuselawyerblog.com/2015/08/nursing-homes-compete-with-lav.html.
23 K. Thomas, "In Race for Medicare Dollars, Nursing Home Care May Lag," *New York Times*, April 14, 2015, https://www.nytimes.com/2015/04/15/business/as-nursing-homes-chase-lucrative-patients-quality-of-care-is-said-to-lag.html, (hereafter cited as "In Race for Medicare Dollars, Nursing Home Care May Lag").

A 2014 report released by the Department of Health and Human Services' Office of the Inspector General stated that nearly one-third of all Medicare patients had experienced "an adverse event or other harm" within approximately 15.5 days of being admitted to a skilled-nursing facility.[24] It reported that physicians who reviewed these findings determined that approximately 59 percent of the adverse events and temporary harm events in all probability could have been prevented. The culprits were mainly attributed to substandard treatment, inadequate resident monitoring, and failure to provide, or a delay in providing, necessary care. The report went on to estimate that Medicare spent $2.8 billion on hospital treatment that resulted from some type of harm in nursing facilities.[25]

The *New York Times* article provides additional information from a 2014 report by Irving Levin Associates, analysts for the senior housing market. Its calculation was that sale prices of nursing homes averaged $76,500 per bed, and this was the second consecutive year of record-breaking prices.[26] In 2016 the reimbursement per bed reached a new high of $99,200, which represented a 15 percent increase from 2015.[27] In spite of the troubling issues with nursing homes, it is clear this is a lucrative

---

24 D. R. Levinson, "Adverse Events in Skilled Nursing Facilities: National Incidence Among Medicare Beneficiaries" Office of Inspector General, accessed September 2017, https://oig.hhs.gov/oei/reports/oei-06-11-00370.pdf, (hereafter cited as "Adverse Events in Skilled Nursing Facilities").

25 "Adverse Events in Skilled Nursing Facilities."

26 "In Race for Medicare Dollars, Nursing Home Care May Lag."

27 "Skilled Nursing Facility Price per Bed Soars to Record, Assisted Living Just Beats Last Year's Record," Irving Levin Associates Inc., accessed February 2017, https://products.levinassociates.com/aboutus/press-releases/prl702scar22/.

business that continues to thrive as evidenced by a 2014 statistic that of the 15,600 nursing homes in the country, 69.8% were for-profit.[28] Indeed, investors and corporations are capitalizing on it at astronomical levels, with no end in sight.

A statement by Bruce Vladeck, who served as director of the Health Care Financing Administration (later renamed the Centers for Medicare & Medicaid Services) in the Clinton administration, expressed the changed effect lobbyists have had on the Medicare program and aptly described the present Medicare environment as changing "from one that provides a legal entitlement to beneficiaries to one that provides a de facto political entitlement to providers."[29]

The emphasis on high reimbursement and competition for Medicare dollars often results in less-than-optimal care in traditional, long-term-care units. The Government Accountability Office (GAO) found that when nursing homes are purchased by for-profit entities, they may—my experience is always—cut staff and other direct-care costs, in order to secure the maximum profit.[30] In 2001 Congress authorized the Department of Health and Human Services to conduct a study on nursing homes and found that 97 percent of nursing homes did not provide the

28 FastStats-Nursing Home Care CDC/National Center for Health Statistics U.S. Department of Health & Human Services Last updated May 3, 2017 accessed October 2017, https://www.cdc.gov/nchs/fastats/nursing-home-care.htm

29 C. Pope, "Medicare's Single-Payer Experience," National Affairs, accessed August 2017, https://www.nationalaffairs.com/publications/detail/medicares-single-payer-experience.

30 "Nursing Homes: Complexity of Private Investment Purchases Demonstrates Need for CMS to Improve the Usability and Completeness of Ownership Data," US Government Accountability Office, accessed August 2017, http://www.gao.gov/assets/320/310562.pdf.

adequate number of nursing care hours per day that were needed to prevent resident harm (e.g., specifically mentioned were pressure sores and weight loss.)[31] The *New York Times* reported on private ownership and quality of nursing-home care in a 2007 investigative article. It focused on more than twelve hundred nursing homes that were purchased by private investment groups. The article analyzed records from the CMS and found that between the years 2000 and 2006, 60 percent of nursing homes that were purchased by private equity firms cut the number of (clinical) registered nurses at times below required legal levels. It also reported, "On average, resident outcomes worsened after private equity groups bought the nursing homes, and their outcomes were worse relative to other nursing homes."[32]

It is unfortunate, after all the years of poor and substandard care and legislation aimed at securing better treatment for our elder citizens, that patients on these units continue to be at the mercy of inexperienced or poorly trained staff and extreme staff shortages resulting in substandard care. These are hallmarks of nursing homes that date back to the early days of the almshouses.

• • •

---

31 "Appropriateness of Minimum Nurse Staffing Ratios in Nursing Homes," Consumer Voice, http://theconsumervoice.org/uploads/files/issues/CMS-Staffing-Study-Phase-II.pdf.

32 C. Duhigg, "At Many Nursing Homes, More Profit and Less Nursing," *New York Times*, September 23, 2007, accessed September 2017, http://www.nytimes.com/2007/09/23/business/23nursing.html?pagewanted=all&_r=0.

Almshouse Population

Despite the trend for nursing homes to incorporate "rehabilitation" in their names, there are facilities where the long-term-care residents have marked similarity to those of days of yore. Beds are filled by a variety of individuals who may otherwise have nowhere else to go. (e.g., alcoholics, drug addicts, mentally/psychologically impaired, and in some cases criminals). Some of these individuals are entirely physically able-bodied (colloquially known by the acronym PAs) and are certainly not in need of the around-the-clock nursing care provided in skilled-nursing facilities.

One facility in which I worked stands out as one of the most egregious examples where these situations exist. A large percentage of the residents were former gang members, murderers, drug dealers, alcoholics, drug addicts, and prostitutes—up to and including a paroled child molester who was on the run and hiding from another state—ranging in age from their mid-twenties to sixty. Many had been part of the prison system that could no longer care for them and other had been homeless. As a matter of fact, some of these residents referred to the facility as a homeless shelter. Among them were those who were entirely able-bodied and who were able to obtain day passes to leave the premises and venture out into the community for undisclosed reasons.

There were many occasions when they would return obviously intoxicated or high on drugs and they would also bring drugs into the facility. At times the smell of marijuana permeated the smoking areas and wafted into the hallways. There were reports of rowdy parties in the evenings, replete with loud, banging music and other behaviors often associated with these situations. Fights would break out, and there were reports of drug dealing in the facility. This was being paid for by tax dollars designated for skilled-nursing care.

All of this happened side by side with older, sick, frail, and confused residents whose home this was meant to be, certainly a far cry from the original intention.

The mixture of the extreme diversity of these two groups was disturbingly reminiscent to the description of the populations in the almshouse years.

Dementia Care versus the "Chandelier Effect"

I attended morning report at a facility with a forty-bed dementia unit, where there were residents with moderate- to advanced-stage dementia. Many of the residents were in wheelchairs, while several others were able to ambulate (walk) independently. The unit was locked, as it is in many facilities, to prevent residents with significant confusion from wandering off into other areas, which could result in unsafe circumstances. The dementia program, as is often the case, consisted of sitting residents in front of a TV with a certified nursing assistant (I) present to watch them. Each time a resident stood up from his or her wheelchair, he or she was told to sit down. There were several residents who were capable of walking and wandered throughout the unit which created a problem for the limited staff. They were also continuously told to sit down.

I suggested making some minor, inexpensive modifications that could address some of these issues. Among them were: painting the unit walls with colors known to be appealing to residents with dementia; applying wall hangings that would engage their attention and focused on providing sensory input (i.e., those they could touch, feel, smell, open, close, and possibly noise activated); ordering plates, cups, and utensils that were brightly colored, which would be more visually appealing by offsetting the bland colors of the puree or ground foods that were prescribed to many residents because of their swallowing difficulties thereby possibly improving food intake; providing food molds so that pureed and ground foods could more closely resemble the food of origin instead of merely looking like scoops on a plate (e.g., pureed/ground fish would be presented in a fish mold or pureed/ground hamburgers or frankfurters would be molded in the shape of the foods they represented); piping in soothing music that would serve to calm those who became easily agitated, and eliminating overhead pages which were loud and startling.

None of these changes were made. Despite the fact that the total cost for these changes probably would not have exceeded a few thousand dollars, cost was raised as the issue. However, the corporation that owned this facility went on to spend over six figures, possibly approaching $150,000 to $200,000, on renovations to the lobby and administrative offices—replete with high-end designer furnishings—as well as to the rehabilitation department and conference room. This is the ultimate example of the chandelier effect. The decor of the patient and resident rooms hardly changed, supplies for patient care remained low, and staffing ratios remained abysmal.

Food Costs versus Quality Care

The dietitian in a facility where I worked said she finally got the costs for meals down to $1.86 per resident, per meal. That calculates out to $5.58 per day, per resident.

A food-service director at another facility told me the budget was $4.65 per resident, per day, and he was told if it went one penny over he would be fired.

Recently a dietitian told me the food cost could be no more than $5.20 per day, per resident, but that number included the costs for supplements. All of these situations were in facilities with a corporate ownership structure that owned a minimum of fifteen nursing homes spanning several states.

A facility that was purchased by a corporation—whose facility ownership burgeoned from eighteen to approximately thirty across several states in the country in just one-and-a-half years—is now substituting powdered cheese for regular cheese in its macaroni and cheese recipe. My colleague said that powdered cheese was not an acceptable protein substitute for regular cheese and wondered how the facility could continue to get away with it.

Food Quality and Portion Size

A facility in which I worked, recently transitioned from not-for-profit ownership to corporate, for-profit ownership. The first changes that became apparent were in the food service department. The director actually told me that the instruction from corporate was that half a million dollars was to be cut from the budget, both in food and staff.

Within a few weeks, the portion sizes of the meals became smaller. Meals were served on each unit in a manner sometimes called country-style dining. On one particular occasion, the server who was unloading the food from her steam cart on the short-term-rehabilitation unit noticed she only had one pan of the main dish, rather than the usual two. She called to the kitchen and asked about the second pan of food. She was told that there would only be one pan available for that meal and that would have to work for all of the patients.

The following day beef stew was the food item for the noon meal. I requested the stew for a patient with whom I was working for consideration of a diet-consistency upgrade. The same server gave me two cubes of beef, approximately one-and-one-half inches in size. I asked her if she was kidding. She informed me that the size of the pan of available food had been reduced by half. Reluctantly, I was given a third piece. In cutting the beef for the patient, I noticed it was extremely hard and I could hardly manage cutting it. This was not what I had seen in the previous few weeks that I had been working at the facility. It was apparent that the quality was already compromised. I thought to myself that if I could hardly cut it, how would patients who may have physical limitations manage cutting, saying nothing of the difficulty they would encounter chewing and swallowing. After the meal was finished, I noticed many patients in that dining room left the meat on their plate and was told the same was true throughout the building.

A few days later I needed to evaluate a resident who was receiving a pu- ree consistency diet to determine if he could manage eating more solid foods. I requested a sandwich snack from the server. What she handed me was shocking. It was a small square with little more than a thin layer of peanut butter and jelly. I could not believe my eyes. It was apparent that the portion size of the sandwich snack was reduced from the typical ½ of a sandwich to ¼ of a sandwich created by cutting the regular sandwich into 4 small squares.

Do these examples demonstrate caring for our elders?

CHAPTER 2

Reimbursement: Insurance Types and Levels

• • •

Medicare Reimbursement

I was present during a recent conversation between a physical-therapy assistant and a rehabilitation-department director. The therapist was advising the director that C. M., a "Medicare A" patient—Med A as it is known colloquially—was not making any progress; therefore, there weren't additional goals to pursue. The director informed the therapist that management expected patients having Medicare A to remain on the therapy program for at least thirty days. The director advised the therapist that he was sure he could report some minor progress for the first two weeks. The second two-week period would bring them near the end of the one-month period at which time he could report the lack of progress and take the patient off the program. In this way, the facility could at least come close to the thirtieth day, whereas if the therapist took the patient off at the two-week mark, it would represent too much of a loss.

Therapy and Ethics

I was completing computer work in an area where a veteran therapist was treating a patient. I heard her say, "This is fraud...I can't do this." I was alarmed by what I heard and turned around; she repeated it, looking straight at me. "This is just fraud; I can't do this. I have to look for a job someplace else."

Maintaining Ultrahigh-RUG Levels

(An explanation of RUG levels and the ultrahigh category of service appears under Medicare A) I was privy to a conversation between a physiatrist and a director of rehabilitation. The physiatrist was stating how it has just become a business—reimbursement and numbers driven. The director's response was to keep the patients going on ultrahigh (referring to the highest level of reimbursement, known as the RUG level) as long as he could.

Overbilling

E. K. was an alert, verbal, gregarious woman at the facility for difficulty walking secondary to a fall and obesity. She particularly enjoyed attending therapy, where she received not only physical and occupational therapies but needed emotional support. She remained at the facility for approximately six months, finally leaving in the early days of June 2015.

Sometime in October 2016, she reached out to one of her former therapists, a colleague with whom I worked closely, to inform her that when she reviewed her insurance information she realized that the facility had actually overcharged her insurance and billed for the entire month of June 2015, despite the fact that she was only there for the first few days of the month. As a result she called the Department of Health to register a complaint, and finally, more than a year later, the facility was being investigated for similar possible charges in other cases.

●　●　●

THE GOVERNMENT ACCOUNTABILITY OFFICE LISTS Medicare as a "high-risk" government program in need of reform; the reason provided is its vulnerability to fraud as well as because of its long-term financial problems.[33],[34] According to the CMS 2013 Report to Congress, fewer than 3 percent of the claims submitted to Medicare each year are manually audited.[35]

MEDICARE

Originally Medicare consisted of only two parts: Medicare Part A and Medicare Part B. It has been expanded to include Medicare Part C and Part D plans as well as ten plans, considered Medicare supplemental plans, under Medigap. The breakdown of Medicare-coverage plans is as follows:

1. Part A—also known as hospital insurance
2. Part B—also known as medical insurance
3. Part C—also known as Medicare Advantage
4. Part D—also known as prescription drug coverage
5. Medigap (Part F)—supplemental Medicare coverage

---

33 "High-Risk Series: An Update," US States Government Accountability Office, accessed September 2017, https://www.gao.gov/assets/240/237065.pdf. accessed September 2017, https://www.gao.gov/assets/240/237065.pdf.

34 "Medicare Fraud and Abuse: DOJ Continues to Promote Compliance with False Claims Act Guidance," US Government Accountability Office, accessed September 2017, www.gao.gov/new.items/d02546.pdf.

35 "Recovery Auditing in Medicare and Medicaid for Fiscal Year 2012," Centers for Medicare & Medicaid Services, accessed September 2017, https://www.cms.gov/Research-Statistics-Data-and-Systems/Monitoring-Programs/Medicare-FFS-Compliance-Programs/Recovery-Audit-Program/Downloads/Report-To-Congress-Recovery-Auditing-in-Medicare-and-Medicaid-for-Fiscal-Year-2012_013114.pdf.

In most cases those who are Part A eligible have paid for their entitlement to coverage under Medicare through the years that the individual or spouse contributed through payroll taxes during their years of employment. Those individuals who are eligible for Medicare A benefits are those over the age of sixty-five, those under sixty-five but with specific disabilities, and any person of any age with end-stage renal disease necessitating dialysis or a kidney transplant.

The following will address the different aspects of these coverages and how they are applied to skilled nursing facilities and rehabilitation centers.

PART A

Medicare A provides recipients with one hundred days of coverage for an inpatient stay, whether it be hospitalization or in a skilled-nursing facility or rehabilitation center, and in some limited circumstances, while at home. The benefit period begins the day of the hospital admission but does not include any days for which a person is admitted for observation. While under observation at the hospital, one is still considered to be an outpatient. Once there is a doctor's order for a hospital admission for a qualifying condition, a three-day, in-hospital stay is required to begin the one hundred Medicare days, as well as for the remaining days beyond the hospitalization to be applied toward a skilled-nursing facility or rehabilitation center stay. The days are applied in totality (e.g., if the patient is hospitalized for thirty days, there would be seventy days remaining for inpatient care at the nursing-home or rehabilitation center).

In order for the skilled-nursing facility or rehabilitation center stay to be covered by the remaining Medicare days following hospitalization, the patient's doctor must have decided that the patient requires daily skilled care either administered by or under direct supervision from skilled nursing or therapy staff. The need for the skilled services must be based on either a medical condition related to the hospital stay or for one that was acquired at the facility during the stay for the medical condition for which the patient was originally hospitalized. Under circumstances where one may only require skilled-rehabilitation services (physical, occupational, or speech therapy), the patient must participate for all the days provided. Refusal could constitute loss of benefits. In the event those services are only provided five or six days a week, the Medicare-benefit days still apply.

Medicare reimburses 100 percent for the first twenty days of an inpatient stay. From day twenty-one through the one hundredth day, the coverage is 80 percent. The remaining 20 percent is an out-of-pocket expense, or copay, for the patient or may be covered by supplementary insurance (e.g., a Medigap plan or other privately held insurance—see discussion that follows).

If the patient is not eligible for discharge once the one hundred days are exhausted, there are a few options available that begin on the 101st day:

1. If the patient has Medicare Part B, that plan continues to cover specific aspects of the cost of the inpatient stay.
2. The patient can pay out of pocket for 100 percent of the charges for the remainder of the stay. (This is referred to as private pay.)

3. If the patient has long-term-care insurance, that will cover the stay.
4. The patient, or the patient's family on the patient's behalf, can apply for one of the following options: Medicaid, Medicaid Managed Care, or Managed Long Term Care (MLTC.

In the event a patient is rehospitalized from the skilled-nursing facility, he or she may return to the same skilled-nursing facility, as long as the institution has an available bed. It should be noted that rehospitalization in the first thirty days following admission is usually frowned upon, and therefore every attempt is made to manage the patient's condition within the facility. Bed-hold policies and reimbursement during hospitalization in SNFs have been studied over the past few years, resulting in recent changes. For example, New York State eliminated its bed-hold policy on April 1, 2017, as a cost-saving measure, but it was reinstated in June 2017. Since repealing bed hold would impact the nursing-home owner's revenue, one can only surmise how it came to be eliminated. (Bed hold is a system whereby the facility continues to be paid a portion of its rate to hold the bed while the patient or resident is hospitalized. Therefore, both the hospital and skilled-nursing facility are being paid for the same person simultaneously. The facility is being paid, while the person is not occupying the bed.)

This is important information one should inquire about upon admission to a facility. The bed-hold policy allows a patient to leave the SNF and return within thirty days without the requisite three-day hospitalization. If there is a break from a skilled-nursing facility of more than thirty days, the required three-day hospitalization period applies in order to qualify for additional care at one of these facilities. In the event one is out of the skilled-nursing facility for at least sixty consecutive days, the maximum one hundred skilled-nursing facility benefit days are renewed.

Prior to 1998 Medicare reimbursed skilled nursing facilities on a fee-for-service system (also known as FFS). In 1998 the CMS changed the reimbursement structure for SNFs to a consolidated billing (CB) system. Under this system the SNF is responsible for providing all covered services to Medicare recipients under a single per-day rate, unless the service has been excluded from this rate.

The covered services include—but are not limited to—bed and board in a semiprivate room; diagnostic x-rays and laboratory work; surgical dressings, splints, and casts; prosthetic devices; leg, arm, back, and neck braces; trusses; artificial limbs, including replacement, adjustment, and repairs; physical, occupational, and speech/language therapy services; and psychological services provided by a clinical social worker, as well as any capital-related costs. (See www.medicare.gov for a complete list of SNF Medicare A-covered services.)

However, there is still variation in the rate, based on the services provided. The highest rates are paid for patients receiving rehabilitation and other specialized services. Those rates are calculated by two factors: the frequency and number of therapy minutes a patient receives based on medical necessity and the skilled-care nursing services needed. The number of therapy minutes and frequency, along with other provided services, are calculated for each patient, which determines the resource utilization group (RUG) category. This becomes the patient's RUG score, which in turn becomes the formula for reimbursement. The more minutes and the greater the number of services provided, the greater the reimbursement rate will be.

In each of the categories the patient must receive that number of minutes as the minimum number in at least five days of a seven-day period. It should be noted that if the therapy minutes exceed the minimum number for a particular category but do not reach the minimum of the following category, the default payment is the minimum number of the previous category. Thus, every effort is made not to exceed the number of minutes in a particular category.

There are facilities that *strictly* adhere to that minimum number and will not exceed it under any circumstances. Other facilities realize that therapy needs to be patient driven and, therefore, should be based on what the patient both needs and can tolerate. Although the directors of rehabilitation departments, whose job it is to calculate, coordinate, and carefully monitor therapy minutes and understand patient need, prefer not to exceed the number by a significant amount, at times it is unavoidable. The breakdown of therapy minutes is as follows:

* **Ultrahigh (the Golden Goose):** 720 minutes—This requires at least two different therapies (physical, occupational, or speech), and at least one therapy must be five days per week; the second can be three days.

- **Very High:** 500 minutes—This requires at least one therapy five days per week, it but can be two or three therapies.
- **High:** 325 minutes—This requires at least one therapy five days per week, but it can be two or three therapies.
- **Medium:** 150 minutes—This requires any one or all three therapies, and the combination of all therapies must be provided at least five days.
- **Low:** 45 minutes—This requires any one or all three therapies to be provided at least three days per week, plus there must be two Minimum Data Set (MDS) areas that provide restorative nursing

Though it seems straightforward and fairly innocuous, there is tremendous manipulation of the minutes to optimize frequency and duration of therapy, so the facility can receive the maximum reimbursement for the maximum number of Medicare days that the patient has available. In most cases when a Medicare patient is admitted, every effort is made to place the person in the *ultrahigh* category; in many of these facilities, this is done almost automatically. However, I personally know of rehabilitation department directors who balk against this practice and base their decisions on what is most clinically appropriate for the patient. In some cases those directors have an adversarial relationship with administration and/or ownership and are pressured to seek maximum reimbursement, regardless of the circumstances.

The Center for Medicare Advocacy (CMA) is fully aware of the problem and reports: "SNFs' manipulation of the therapy classification to which they assign residents resulted in 'excessive payments.'" In 2012 the CMS made several attempts to readjust the Medicare reimbursement rates. The purpose of the reduction was specifically intended to focus on the overpayment of therapy-related reimbursement.[36]

At the time RUG levels were introduced, there were forty-four categories that determined rates; that jumped to fifty-three in 2006 and finally to sixty-six categories for fiscal year 2011. The latest increased to include both rehabilitation and the extensive services categories. One CMS statistic indicates 92 percent of all Medicare residents are assigned to a rehabilitation category.[37] Because a facility receives the highest reimbursement for Medicare A patients, these patients have become the most coveted. This has been the impetus for skilled nursing facilities becoming rehabilitation centers and revamping or renovating their facilities for high-end appeal. This has also created the desire on the part of some companies to pressure service providers to inflate the scores so that they can receive an even higher Medicare reimbursement.

The Department of Justice found just cause for two such claims. In November 2013 the Ensign Group Inc., a California-based company that operates nursing homes across the western

---

36 "SNF Therapy Payment Models Base Year Final Summary," Centers for Medicare & Medicaid Services, accessed October 2016, https://www.cms.gov/Medicare/Medicare-Fee-for-Service-Payment/SNFPPS/Downloads/Summary_Report_20140501.pdf.

37 "Medicare Reimbursement for Skilled Nursing Facilities Remains High for 2012 Despite Reductions in Overpayments," Center for Medicare Advocacy, accessed October 2016, http://www.medicareadvocacy.org/medicare-reimbursement-for-skilled-nursing-facilities-remains-high-for-2010-despite-reductions-in-overpayments/, (hereafter cited as "Medicare Reimbursement for Skilled Nursing Facilities Remains High").

United States, paid $48 million in federal fines to settle charges that the group submitted Medicare claims either exaggerating patients' rehabilitation needs or providing unnecessary rehabilitation services.[38] Extendicare Health Services Inc., a large Canadian company, and its subsidiary, Progressive Step Corporation, paid $38 million dollars to settle claims for both. In the latter case the company was also required to enter into a five-year agreement to assure chain-wide corporate integrity.[39]

There are some facilities that are moving to take only Medicare patients and totally moving away from the long-term-care model. These facilities do everything in their power to attract Medicare patients in an effort to reap the most profits. In addition, there are also efforts to either exhaust a patient's allotted Medicare days, which may result in keeping patients in a program beyond what is actually clinically appropriate, or to delay a discharge in order to achieve the projected therapy minutes for the projected RUG category before the designated assessment reference date. (More information as it pertains to assessment reference dates may be found in the chapter on MDS.)

---

38 "Nursing Home Operator to Pay $48 Million to Resolve Allegations that Six California Facilities billed for Unnecessary Therapy," United States Department of Justice, accessed September 2017 US Department of Justice, accessed September 2017, https://www.justice.gov/opa/pr/nursing-home-operator-pay-48-million-resolve-allegations-six-california-facilities-billed.

39 "Extendicare Health Services Inc. Agrees to Pay $38 Million to Settle False Claims Act Allegations Relating to the Provision of Substandard Nursing Care and Medically Unnecessary Rehabilitation Therapy," United States Department of Justice, accessed September 2017 https://www.justice.gov/opa/pr/extendicare-health-services-inc-agrees-pay-38-million-settle-false-claims-act-allegations.

Part B

Medicare Part B covers a variety of services not covered under Part A. *Some* of these are diagnostic lab tests, X-rays, surgery, doctors' visits and other hospital outpatient services, ambulance transportation, rehabilitation services (e.g., physical, occupational, and speech therapy), some home health care and equipment that is deemed to be medically necessary (such as wheelchairs or walkers, whether purchased or rented), orthotic or prosthetic devices, and surgical dressings or wound treatment. Medicare Part B also extends this coverage for those who have enrolled to patients and residents in nursing homes.

Medical necessity is what is needed to diagnose or treat a medical condition according to accepted and standard medical practice. It also covers preventive measures when delivered to prevent illness (e.g., inoculations for the flu) or to detect illness at an early stage (e.g., cancer screenings).

There is a cost for Part B coverage that is paid as a monthly premium. However, if the enrollee did not sign up for Part B coverage when first eligible for Part A, the premium will increase up to 10 percent for each twelve-month period that the person could have had Part B but did not because he or she did not enroll upon initial eligibility. This increased cost continues as long as the beneficiary receives Part B benefits. There is also a yearly deductible that must be met each year before the Medicare benefits begin. In specific cases an enrollee may apply to the state for assistance with the premium and deductible. These premium and deductible rates may change in January each year.

Most Part B services provided to nursing-home residents who are not in a Part A-covered stay are not subject to consolidated billing requirements. Instead each service provider may submit a separate claim to Medicare for each service rendered.

PART C (MEDICARE ADVANTAGE PLAN [MAP])

Medicare Part C was established as part of the Balanced Budget Act of 1997 (BBA) that went into effect in January 1999. At that time it was known as the Medicare + Choice (M+C) program. The purpose was to offer lower-cost coverage beyond the Medicare Parts A and B plan via public or private companies that would be able to provide more options by contracting with Medicare. These options included health-maintenance organizations (HMOs), preferred-provider organizations (PPOs), medical-savings accounts (MSA), provider-sponsored organizations (PSOs), private fee for service (PFFS), and plans affiliated with religious organizations (also known as fraternal-benefit-society plans).

There were many problems associated with the M+C plan, due to the limited number of plans offered to those living in rural areas, large discrepancies in payments among geographic areas, and many plans preferring to leave the M+C program altogether. Thus in 2003 the federal government legislated the Medicare Modernization Act (MMA) that replaced the M+C Program with what is now known as the Medicare Advantage Plan (MAP). The intention of this new program was not only to address the aforementioned problems with the M+C Program but also to introduce the Part D benefit plan. The CMS set forth proposed regulations for this new plan in August 2004. The regulations were finalized on January 28, 2005, and the program was implemented beginning March 22, 2005.

Plans that fall in the Medicare Advantage category are issued by private insurance companies that contract with and are approved by Medicare. Medicare pays these private insurance companies a fixed monthly fee, and they in turn cover medical costs as stipulated by Medicare Part C. They provide all the Medicare Part A in-hospital stay coverage as well as the Part B medical insurance coverage, but there are usually added benefits that these plans offer (e.g., vision, dental, and hearing).

Some plans also offer coverage for prescription drugs and are known as a Medicare Advantage Prescription Drug Plan. The fundamental difference with these plans, as opposed to Medicare Parts A and B, is that despite the word "Medicare" they function very similarly to traditional medical insurance companies, because a private insurance company underwrites them.

Some noted restrictions with them is that one may be limited to seeing specific in-network doctors or going to specific network hospitals, and a referral may be needed in order to see a specialist. Furthermore, the out-of-pocket and deductible expenses of these plans may vary—they may be higher or lower than traditional Medicare and dependent on the plan purchased and services utilized. For the most part, there is a yearly maximum out-of-pocket expense; once that amount has been reached, there is no additional cost for any services one might need. These specifics vary from plan to plan and are subject to change on a yearly basis.

In order to qualify for Medicare Part C, one must live in the service area of the plan desired, have Medicare Parts A and B coverage, and not have end-stage renal disease. (There may be a few exceptions to this last qualifier.)

The different forms of MAPs include the following:

1. HMO
2. PPO
3. PFFS
4. Special needs plans (SNPs)
5. HMO point-of-service (HMOPOS)

One should inquire about the pros and cons of each plan prior to enrolling, as each plan may have different aspects that may or may not be applicable to a nursing home or rehabilitation center stay. For example, an important consideration is that because these companies contract with Medicare to carry the MAP on a yearly basis, they can choose not to renew their contract. It should also be noted that the premiums, benefits, and copayments are subject to change each year. There are also restrictions for reenrollment.

One can always enroll when first becoming eligible, but normally the plan can only be changed once a year during what is known as the *annual election period,* which runs from October 15 through December 7. (Under certain circumstances one may qualify for a special election period.) If for some reason a person wants to disenroll and return to the original Medicare plan, that period extends from January 1 through February 14 each year. This is known as the *disenrollment period.*

According to www.medicare.gov, there are fifty-five million people participating in the traditional Medicare program who purchase supplemental coverage for the remaining 20 percent or other out-of-pocket expenses. A substantial number of people, albeit a much smaller number when compared to the fifty-five million, have purchased private coverage through Medicare Part C or MAP.[40]

PART D (PRESCRIPTION DRUG BENEFIT)

Medicare Part D was introduced with the passage of MMA and went into effect in January 2006. The purpose was to help defray the high costs of prescription drugs and the associated insurance premiums for Medicare enrollees.

Those individuals interested in purchasing coverage under Part D must already be enrolled in the Medicare Part A and Part B programs. There are two types of Part D plans, both of which are administered by private insurance companies. The prescription drug plan (PDP) is a straight Medicare Part D plan. The second type is the Part C plan (i.e., the MAP) and covers all the hospital and medical services covered under Medicare Parts A and B as well as the additional services described in that section, including prescription drugs.

---

40 *Wikipedia*, s.v. "Medicare (United States)," accessed September 2017, https://en.wikipedia.org/wiki/Medicare_(United_States).

Out-of-pocket expenses and copays are not covered at the same rate under the plans, giving enrollees choices of drugs in a particular category or for a particular condition or ailment (e.g., name brand or generic). One should not automatically assume the generic formulation of a particular drug will be less expensive. The cost is based on a complicated formula manipulated by pharmaceutical companies. It is always best to ask specifics about out-of-pocket and total-drug cost for any particular prescription drug item.

In order to receive the subsidies that defray the cost of prescription drugs, one must participate in either a Medicare Part C or D program. An individual can enroll in one of three ways: (1) via an insurance broker from a private insurance company that contracts with Medicare (as in the MAP), (2) with an individual insurance broker, or (3) in an exchange run by the CMS. The same rights regarding prescription plan subsidies are afforded to all enrollees, regardless of the way they choose to enroll.

There are specific enrollment periods throughout the year; at present the annual enrollment period lasts from October 15 to December 7. However, senior citizens who fall into a low-income category and who also receive Social Security Extra Help/Low-Income Subsidy—as well as many of those considered to be in a middle-income bracket who are enrolled in state-pharmaceutical-assistance programs—can choose a different plan or alternately enroll and drop Part C or Part D as often as once a month as the situation dictates. Other special enrollment circumstances may apply.

If a Medicare beneficiary wishes to enroll at a later date because he or she did not enroll when first eligible, the person will pay a late-enrollment penalty. This is also known as a premium surtax. This penalty is equal to 1 percent of the national premium index times the number of full calendar months that the person was eligible but not enrolled in Part D and did not have creditable coverage through another source (e.g., an employer or veterans receiving benefits through the Veterans Administration).

MEDIGAP (PLAN F)

Medigap is merely a supplemental insurance for Medicare that is sold by private insurance companies to fill the gap between what Medicare covers and does not cover. It can help pay copayments, coinsurance, and deductibles and *may* also, depending on the policy, provide coverage when traveling outside of the United States. Medigap coverage begins after traditional Medicare pays its covered portion. It is not a substitute for Medicare; it is solely gap coverage. There are ten types of Medigap plans, and each state usually classifies the different plans with letters—: A, B, C, D, F, G, K, L, M, and N—although the insurance companies in each state may not carry all ten plans.

It is important to note that a plan ascribed with a specific letter carries the same benefits across state lines, although each insurance company has its own rate structure. Massachusetts, Minnesota, and Wisconsin have different methods for standardizing their plans. For more information about insurance coverage or to answer questions about dropping coverage, visit www.medicare.gov, www.medicareproviders.net, or www.medicare16.org.

Medigap Essentials to Know:

1. One must already have Medicare Parts A and B.
2. There is a monthly insurance premium payable to the private insurance company that issues the policy. This is in addition to Part B premiums.
3. One can apply for <u>Medigap</u> insurance if already enrolled in a Medicare Advantage Plan (MAP), but you must <u>disenroll</u> from the MAP prior to the beginning of the Medigap policy.
4. <u>Medigap</u> policies apply to each individual. Spouses must purchase their own <u>Medigap</u> policy.
5. The company from whom the policy is purchased must be licensed in the state where the person enrolling resides.
6. There is a policy-renewal guarantee for <u>Medigap</u> policies, regardless of medical condition, as long as the premiums are paid and current.
7. <u>Medigap</u> policies, as of January 2006, do not include prescription drugs. Prescription drug plans are covered under Medicare Part D.
8. <u>Medigap</u> open-enrollment period begins six months after individual turns sixty-five and six months after the individual enrolls in Part B.

It is important to note that during the open-enrollment period, the status of one's health cannot be a factor when issuing the policy. Policy rates can only be based on age and other demographic considerations. Therefore it would be prudent to enroll during this period—especially if one has health concerns or issues. There is, however, a waiting period where preexisting conditions are concerned. This means an insurance company may refuse to pay for health-care expenses incurred related to a preexisting condition, which can continue for up to six months maximum after the policy has been signed. After that time period, payment for that condition resumes.

Medicare Part F is considered to be the preferred and most comprehensive of all the Medicare supplemental plans. This is because Medicare is considered to have nine gaps in coverage, and the Part F supplemental plan covers each. An enrollee choosing this option would pay Part A and Part B coverage, Part D prescription coverage, and the Part F Medigap Supplemental Coverage. The enrollee would essentially not pay any additional charges for medical treatment or services. This option covers the Part A deductible and coinsurance, the Part B deductible and excess charges, and the skilled-nursing facility coinsurance up to one hundred days, as well as providing an additional 365 days of hospital coverage, bringing the total of 100 percent covered hospitalization days to 515. If traveling abroad one would be responsible for the first $250 and 20 percent coinsurance for any emergency medical treatment.

An additional benefit is that if the enrollee is on Social Security, the premium can be deducted (as it also can for Medicare Parts A, B, and D).

Managed Care (HMOs)

An HMO is a type of insurance plan that provides health coverage but limits the coverage to doctors and facilities that contract with that particular insurance carrier.

The only exception would be a health situation that required emergency care, urgent care outside of the service area, or dialysis treatment, if one is outside of the service area. As a result of these contracted relationships, the insured often cannot continue with a doctor or specialist with whom he or she has had a relationship over a period of time.

There are HMO plans that will allow the enrollee to go out of the network for particular services, although the premium for such a policy would in most cases be higher. These plans are known as HMO with a point-of-service (POS) option. There may be restrictions in terms of where an insured works or resides in relation to the insurance carrier.

An important focus of HMOs is prevention and wellness. Most HMO plans also provide prescription drug coverage. In these types of plans, the insured pays a fixed monthly fee to the insurance company that is not dependent on the type or level of service required for a particular medical situation or condition. Nursing homes and rehabilitation centers do not accept all HMO plans and, therefore, cannot accept admissions from companies with whom they do not have a contract.

In addition, the facility contracts with the HMO at particular levels of service. Since HMO plans pay facilities a set rate based on the contract as well as the type of plan purchased by the beneficiary, the facility does not receive higher rates for patients, regardless of the extent of services they receive and whether or not they receive rehabilitation services. Since frequency and duration of treatment are not considerations, this may reflect negatively on the HMO patient's treatment plan. The patient with HMO coverage usually receives less therapy in both frequency and duration, oftentimes for the same condition as the Medicare counterpart who is, at the same time, receiving maximum therapy minutes and frequency.

Furthermore, patients are often seen in concurrent or group treatments, yet they are billed individually. This is in direct contrast to Medicare standards and practice. (See example below.) It is this writer's contention that HMOs should adopt the same stringent requirements for individualized treatment as Medicare. Additionally, therapists are also required to write frequent notes for the HMO—often weekly—to justify rehabilitation services. Continuation in therapy is at the discretion of the reviewer at the HMO office. There are many instances of denial that can be, and usually are, appealed with no guarantee of a favorable outcome. In many cases facilities do not desire to take patients with HMO coverage.

Here is an example of therapy services delivered and billed in three ways:

- *Individual therapy*, which is a one-on-one session
- *Group therapy*, where one therapist works with several residents on the same task
- *Concurrent therapy*, where one therapist works with several residents on different tasks but at the same time

Medicare rules have become more stringent in this area. Up until several years ago, the most common practice, especially for occupational and physical therapy, was to work with several residents at the same time but to bill each of them for the full number of minutes (e.g., one could be working with three patients at the same time for forty-five minutes, and the therapist would bill each patient for the full forty-five minutes). That changed several years ago, when Medicare eliminated the practice of treating patients in group or concurrent sessions and billing them on an individual basis. In the event a patient had to be seen in a group or concurrent session, the minutes would have to be divided among the patients in the group. (So, in this same example, each patient would be billed for fifteen minutes.) Since the frequency and duration of therapy minutes for Medicare patients help determine their RUG category, which counts toward the reimbursement that the facility receives, they would most likely not be seen in group or concurrent sessions.

The HMO patient, for whom the facility receives one contracted rate no matter the number of services he or she receives, is at a distinct disadvantage. This issue of individual or concurrent therapy treatment is not only critical for the patient but has tremendous implications for therapists who are now pressured toward 100 percent productivity. Rehabilitation-department directors, under pressure from their organization superiors and in an effort to maximize productivity and demonstrate department profitability, can schedule physical and occupational therapists for over 100 percent productivity in a day. While this does not seem to make logical sense—How can a person be more productive than the number of hours he or she is working?—it makes sense monetarily, if one considers the calculation for therapy according to HMO standards versus Medicare standards. Because the treating therapist can treat several HMO patients at one time, yet bill them individually, the therapist can achieve a higher productivity than the number of hours worked. This is not only a troubling ethical issue for therapists and their professional organizations, but it should also be troubling for the HMO as well as regulatory bodies that oversee the workforce.

In 2009 the CMS found that 28.26 percent of therapy conducted in skilled nursing facilities was delivered concurrently. That translated into the facility billing Medicare as if each resident received 100 percent of the therapist's attention.[41] As a result, for the fiscal year 2010, CMS initiated placing limitations on the facilities' use of concurrent therapy and changed the way it could be applied. In this new paradigm, if therapy was provided to two individuals simultaneously, the therapy time

---

41 "Medicare Reimbursement for Skilled Nursing Facilities Remains High."

had to be split and billed to each person accordingly, requiring allocation of concurrent therapy time between residents and limiting concurrent therapy to two residents. An example of this problematic situation appears in an article entitled "Under Pressure" and published in the *ASHA Leader* magazine.[42] The article addresses the issue of the expectations and pressure for high productivity in skilled nursing facilities and the effect this has on patient care and service delivery. The writer explains that the nature of Medicare's reimbursement system is the driving force behind the high-productivity demands for speech/language pathologists and occupational and physical therapists. In that paradigm only actual treatment time with the patient is reimbursable. This excludes evaluation time to determine the need for therapy or the course of treatment, as an evaluation is not considered treatment.

I have several personal experiences that exemplify this situation. One that is particularly outstanding is when I was called to a facility to evaluate a patient but was asked if I was going to put the person on a program prior to my evaluation. I informed the director of nurses who asked that I had no way of knowing until I had completed my assessment. The response was that the facility was not reimbursed for evaluation time, so unless I was going to put the person on the program, she would rather not have me do the assessment. I informed her that I in no way could determine that beforehand any more than a doctor's office could tell her when she called for an

---

42 M. Cutter, "Under Pressure," *The ASHA Leader,* accessed April 2017, leader.pubs. asha.org/issue.aspx?issueid=930256, (hereafter cited as "Under Pressure").

appointment whether or not medication would be prescribed prior to the examination by the doctor. That response made sufficient sense for me to receive the go-ahead to evaluate the patient.

Medicare instituted the concept of actual treatment time for the purpose of reimbursement in 1998 as a stopgap measure against skyrocketing costs. Because therapy minutes are calculated to determine the individual's all-important RUG level, any time not spent with the patient is also not reimbursable. Aspects that are not reimbursable include consultation with other therapists or staff, doctors, or dietitians; care-plan meetings; any family consultation or education in which the patient is not present; documentation; and reports. Time that is not billable includes walking from one patient to the next, elevator waiting or riding time, or even a bathroom break.

While the intention behind Medicare's methodology may have seemed reasonable and sound, unfortunately the purveyors of the skilled nursing facility business have used this methodology to pressure therapists approaching—and in some cases exceeding, as with HMOs—100 percent productivity, all for the purposes of ensuring that they receive the maximum reimbursement for the least expenditure. Every minute of staff time must be accounted for and be reimbursable.

I was recently told that lawyers bill for thinking about a client and that I can do the same. Most recently I heard a rehabilitation department director tell occupational therapy (OT) and physical therapy (PT) staff that they should consider educating their patient or resident while riding in the elevator as part of the session. However, that director—besides espousing a practice that is totally misguided—was not considering that it would be a serious violation of the Health Insurance Portability and Accountability Act (HIPAA) and would certainly constitute a violation of the patient's privacy, especially if there were any other individuals in or around the elevator at the time.

I know this director, as many others, are under tremendous pressure from superiors to achieve the highest staff-to-patient productivity ratios. These are not isolated examples. The *ASHA Leader* article cites a 2012 Urban Institute report that was issued to the Medicare Payment Advisory Commission that stated, "The system did not accurately pay for non-therapy ancillary services [and] encouraged facilities to provide therapy services for financial, not clinical, reasons."[43]

The July 2014 issue of *PT in Motion*, a magazine published by the American Physical Therapy Association, reported: "PTs and PTAs need not just have the ethical courage to stand up for what is right, but also tools and resources to fortify them to engage vigorously and effectively in the dialogue and negotiations with administrators/employers and consultants who are pressuring [them] to adopt productivity measures or practices that may represent sincere but archaic or misguided notions of the nature and role of PT practice."[44]

---

43 "Under Pressure," 36–44.

44 "From the House of Delegates: Help in Responding to 'Productivity' Issues on Its Way," *PT in Motion*, July 9, 2014, accessed February 2017, http://www.apta.org/PTinMotion/NewsNow/2014/7/9/HoDProductivity/.

MEDICAID MANAGED CARE (MMC)

A fundamental difference between Medicare and Medicaid is that to enroll in Medicare, one must be sixty-five years or older.

Medicaid, on the other hand, is a program that is not age dependent. It is a health-care program funded by the federal government but run by individual states to assist those with low income to pay for long-term medical or custodial care. Adults of any age may apply, as long as they meet the income restrictions and other guidelines and are residents or citizens of the United States. The benefits can extend to the family or dependents of the applicant as well as to those with specific disabilities.

Individual states have their own guidelines regarding eligibility, and they are also free to determine whether or not they will participate in the program. If one does not already have Medicaid when hospitalized, the social worker of that institution can assist with the application process. If one is already in a nursing home or rehabilitation center, has exhausted Medicare or other coverage benefits, and is eligible for skilled nursing or long-term-care placement, the social worker can also assist with the application process. If one wants to determine eligibility in advance of hospitalization, this information can be found by visiting the Health Insurance Marketplace website or www. healthcare.gov to locate the individual state's Medicaid agency.

In 2010 President Barack Obama signed what is known as the Affordable Care Act (ACA), expanding Medicaid coverage to legal residents and US citizens making up to 133 percent of the poverty line in those states that participate in the program. States can continue to receive Medicaid funding whether or not they agreed to participate in this expanded coverage. As of January 2016, in addition to the District of Columbia, thirty-one states have agreed to participate in the expanded coverage. (See appendix for the list of states.)

The impending repeal of the ACA will most probably impact Medicaid coverage for many residents and citizens. The verdict is yet to be determined as to how this will play out for those in need.

Medicaid Managed Care (MMC) is a system that was devised to provide health care with increased focus on cost management, quality of care, utilization of services, and treatment outcomes. This accomplished by organizations known as managed care organizations (MCOs) contracting with state Medicaid agencies. Fees are established and capped for each covered individual on a monthly basis, thereby reducing the cost of the program to the individual state. There are efforts by some states to more closely examine ways to ensure improved quality of care for those with chronic or complicated medical conditions as well as to incorporate incentives for achieving patient goals and higher standards of quality of care.

Some Medicaid programs offer an FFS system where each health-care provider is paid a preset amount for each service provided, whether it be a doctor's visit, test, or procedure. These rates also apply to services provided within the skilled-nursing facility or rehabilitation center. Therefore, any time a specialist would visit or provide service to a resident, he or she would bill Medicaid (e.g., ophthalmology, optometry, podiatry, dentistry, audiology, etc.). This would also include any visits to specialists outside of the facility. However, because of the limited amount paid to specialists, it is often difficult for a facility to find specialists to either visit the facility to provide service or to see residents in their office. Oftentimes facilities try to disenroll patients or residents from MMC plans because the reimbursement rate is less than what the facility would receive from the straight Medicaid benefits program. Medicaid managed care plans also allow individuals to remain in their home and receive at-home or community based services for longer periods of time. However, if a person's medical or physical status becomes more serious, he or she may eventually find themselves admitted to a nursing home, Not all facilities accept all MMC plans. Therefore, in some situations an individual may have to apply for an MMC plan accepted by that particular facility.

Long-Term-Care Insurance Plans

The purpose of long-term-care insurance is to provide coverage for long-term-care services and corresponding supportive needs that may include personal and custodial care often referred to as activities of daily living (ADLs), which include bathing, dressing, or eating. The insurance covers that care whether it be in a long-term-care facility, the home, a community organization, or other type of facility. Policies are issued by private insurance companies. Reimbursement amounts are stipulated on a daily basis that an individual will select when purchasing the policy. As with any other type of insurance, it is best to shop around for the kinds of coverage being considered as well as the range of care options and benefits that each policy will provide. It is undeniable that these are difficult decisions to make when a person cannot foresee what his or her needs will look like in advancing years or conditions.

Costs of policies will depend on a variety of factors:

1. Age when purchasing the policy
2. The maximum daily amount the policy will cover
3. The maximum duration of the policy (in days or years)
4. Whether or not optional benefits will be purchased (i.e., accounting for an increase with inflation)

Many long-term-care insurance policies have a specific length of time for which they will pay. For example, there are policies that will pay up to two to five years and others that will continue to pay for the lifetime regardless of cost. Most policies have some kind of limit attached to them. The lifetime maximum policy amount is calculated by multiplying the maximum amount per day by the number of coverage days. Be advised that long-term-care insurance policies do not significantly differ from any other insurance policy and rates may increase over time, which may be simply an inflationary adjustment. It is worth considering requesting information on the company's premium rate history.

In the event an individual's health is already compromised or is in decline, this may be considered a preexisting condition that may exclude the person from purchasing a long-term-care policy. However, there may be plans that may allow the purchase of limited coverage or coverage for a higher premium amount.

More information on long-term-care insurance can be found at AARP.org, where there is an article entitled "Understanding Long-Term Care Insurance: Basics of Health Care Insurance Coverage."

• • •

Unrealistic Productivity Trends

I met the new director of the rehabilitation department where I was working. We introduced ourselves to each other, and then he proceeded to say, "I expect 90 to 100 percent productivity. I have three corporate people above me that I have to answer to, and if productivity falls below 90 percent, I'll get yelled at and have to explain it. I also need at least fifteen residents picked up for CMI."

There were no questions about my experience, how long I had been working there, or whether there were any issues that might need to be addressed within the facility. His introduction to me was similar to the way he introduced himself to the other therapists in the department.

Productivity at 100 percent is not possible. We are not robots, and neither are the patients or residents we treat. They are sick or impaired in some way; many of them are older or frail, and sometimes they are confused. How can 100 percent productivity be achieved when patients don't feel well, need to use the bathroom in the middle of a session, or have trouble getting up on a particular day? How do we account for the time to transport patients from one floor to another or even from their room located on the same floor as the therapy department? There is also the staff shortage situation to consider which results in patients who are late getting up in the morning and who are not ready for therapy on time. Meal service might be running a little behind schedule, or there might be an out-of-facility doctor's appointment or an in-house doctor's consultation.

Therapists are declaring 100 percent is fraudulent. (I also declare it is both unethical and fraudulent.) Yet this is the trend: numbers, numbers, numbers, resulting in dollars, dollars, dollars. The director didn't care how we got it, just as long as we got it. Therapists were already talking of leaving, and the new director hadn't even started.

Job versus Productivity

A colleague told me she went for an interview at a facility where the director of the re-habilitation department told her the expected productivity was 100 percent. She told me her response was, "thank you for the offer but I am not willing to commit fraud."

Several months later she found herself working at a facility where the same company for whom the previous director worked, took over the rehabilitation department. The therapist met with the regional director regarding her concerns over the unrealistic productivity demands. She told me the regional director told her she should learn to type faster.

At the aforementioned facility therapists are pressured to write their notes during the patient's therapy session in order to meet the high productivity de-mands. It is based on the fact that if the patient is present during note writing, the therapist can bill the required therapy minutes. However, the patient is certainly getting shortchanged. Each day I observe patients sitting idle watching therapists busy typing away on their computers. Every few minutes the therapist turns to the patient to see if he or she has completed a required activity or exercise, ask a question, or to instruct them to do another task, after which they return bus-ily to their note writing. Productivity remains high. The therapist is billing for the required minutes maintaining the company's financial expectations; however, the patient is definitely getting shortchanged in terms of their therapy treatment time.

It has been suggested that I also use an iPad to write notes during my ses-sions. I have refused questioning the ethics and presenting the argument that it is counterintuitive to speech and communications where face to face interactions are integral to the process.

For the most part, the therapists feel as though they are trapped. They fear if they don't acquiesce and meet the demands, they will be out of a job and re-placed. There is always someone who will take the job and "follow orders".

Therapy Need versus Reimbursement

During a care-plan meeting that I was attending for a stroke patient, the daughter asked the director of the rehabilitation department about massage for her mother's shoulder on the affected side. She said she had heard that massage had been helpful in patients' return of function in the affected arm. The director informed her that the facility did not offer massage.

Back in the rehabilitation department, I questioned the director about the massage. In almost every other facility in which I had worked, occupational therapists regularly massaged the shoulders or knees of patients for whom they thought it would be beneficial. I stated that if massage would be helpful in facilitating return of function, a few minutes couldn't hurt. He reiterated it was not reimbursable; therefore, they would not do it. if the patient wanted massage, she should hire a massage therapist.

Marketing

I was speaking with a director of admissions about her marketing role, in which she conducted tours for families. The facility had new corporate ownership that had been cutting staff hours, reducing availability of supplies, and serving less-satisfying food, resulting in many complaints from both families and staff members. Her comment to me about the ownership during one conversation was, "They don't give a rat's ass about the facility or the patients." In another conversation she said, "I have a problem selling shit." During the latter part of that conversation, she went on to say, "At least I know the rehabilitation department is excellent, so when I take families to see it, I know I'm telling them the truth when I say what a great team it is and talk about the great work they do." She went on to say that "everyone has complaints about these facilities."

Exhausting Medicare Days

I was seeing a patient for appropriate diet consistency at a facility in which I was covering for a vacationing therapist. A. G. was a pleasant, alert, and well-spoken gentleman who was recovering after a fall. He informed me he had already been at the facility for several weeks and was walking without difficulty. He was sure he was ready to return home and already had the necessary services and equipment in place prior to being hospitalized.

A. G. complained that he asked about discharge on several occasions and felt he was being "strung along" so that the facility could use up his Medicare days. He said he felt "stuck" because there was no one who could advocate for him. He had additional concerns about the consequences if some other medical situation arose shortly after he returned home and his Medicare days had been exhausted.

I felt terrible about the situation. I tried to be as supportive as possible and assured A. G. I would mention it to the director of the rehabilitation department. However, as a visiting therapist, there were limits to the extent of my advocacy.

Prospective Payment System

• • •

Therapy Minutes and RUG Categories

I was seated next to the director of a rehabilitation department when a patient (V. M.) arrived in the office to speak with him. The patient said he told the occupational and physical therapists that he did not want to participate in therapy on Saturdays, but they continued to force him to do it. On the previous weekend, he said the therapists dragged him to participate in therapy even though he had told them he was sick. He found out after the weekend that he had pneumonia. He went on to explain to the director that even when he was at home he stayed in bed and rested on Saturdays.

The director explained to the patient that his Medicare insurance had him slotted to participate in therapy six days per week, and if he did not participate, his Medicare might not continue covering the cost of his stay in the facility. This was not the case at all. The fact was that V. M. was scheduled for six days a week of therapy so that he would attain the necessary 720 minutes for the ultrahigh-RUG category, (sixty minutes each of physical therapy and occupational therapy each day for six days) thereby ensuring the facility would receive the maximum reimbursement. The therapists are instructed to complete the required therapy minutes under any circumstances. Many times the patient's wishes are not a consideration in that formula.

RUG Level and Therapy Minutes versus Discharge

I attended the discharge plan meeting with my friend who was on the short-term rehabilitation unit of a facility following hip surgery. He had been there for two weeks, and being a strong, physically active, professional man, he was eager to return home with the understanding that he would continue to receive physical therapy at a local outpatient clinic. The meeting took place on a Tuesday, and he informed the "team" that he wanted to leave on Friday. The social worker responded that his request was not possible, as the facility had several discharges already planned for that day and could not plan for another. I interjected that since my friend had therapy on Sunday and was scheduled to receive therapy every day in the week, including Friday morning, he would achieve the required number of therapy minutes and, therefore, could be discharged Friday afternoon. The social worker immediately excused herself. Upon returning she reported that indeed the facility could accommodate his request to leave Friday.

● ● ●

Included in the Balanced Budget Act of 1997 was Section 4432(a), which addressed and changed a critical reimbursement component for those Medicare patients receiving skilled-nursing facility services during the portion of their stay that was covered by Medicare Part A insurance. Prior to passage of this bill, facilities were paid on what was considered to be reasonable costs and a low-volume rate. The passage of this legislation changed the reimbursement structure to what is now known as the Prospective Payment System (PPS).

Brief History and Synopsis

Research to revamp the reimbursement system for nursing-home facilities was actually initiated in the 1970s for two reasons: to fine-tune the payment system and to improve quality of care. The resulting system was based in part on work conducted by several states that developed a system that came to be known as a Case-Mix payment system. Case Mix is a classification system in which the care offered to an individual resident is classified into categories based on the intensity of the care and services provided. It considers diagnoses, conditions, treatments, and assistance with activities of daily living (ADLs). Residents are then classified into resource utilization groups based on the likelihood they will utilize specific resources.

This system was initially used as a method of reimbursement for Medicaid nursing-home recipients. Currently the Case-Mix methodology is the basis for the PPS for both skilled nursing facilities and swing-bed hospitals. While Case Mix is the basis for the PPS, with recipients receiving services in a skilled-nursing facility as part of a Medicare Part A covered stay, there are an increasing number of states using the Case-Mix system as a formula for calculating Medicaid reimbursement. Further discussion of Case Mix for Medicaid recipients will be undertaken in the chapter on Case-Mix Index.

The Case-Mix system takes into account the different levels of care provided to the varied types of cases within the facility—hence the term "Case Mix"—as well as wage differences of varying geographic regions in the country. (This latter consideration was based on what is known as the hospital-wage index.) In addition, routine and ancillary services and the facility's capital-related expenses were accounted for in the reimbursement formula.

The rates were determined through what may seem to be a confusing method. It uses an estimate for the cost of services paid to beneficiaries covered by Medicare Part B but paid during that portion of their stay that was covered by Medicare Part A. A national average was then taken of the aggregate data for facilities in both urban and rural areas. That average facilitated a federal standard per diem rate that took into account the Case Mix and wage adjustments for that area. The Case-Mix adjustment is a classification system based on the RUG score, which is determined from a resident-assessment instrument as well as weighted information based on staff-time information. The resident-assessment instrument uses what is known as the Minimum Data Set 3.0 (MDS). Daily per-patient rates are based on what is colloquially known as four buckets of expenses that include the following:

1. Direct costs consisting of clinical, therapeutic, and supportive care expenses (e.g., nursing staff salaries) as well as the Case-Mix score
2. Indirect costs (housekeeping, laundry, dietary, administration, utilities, and insurance)
3. Capital costs (interest and depreciation for approved capital expenses)
4. Noncomparable costs (staff or services beyond basic direct costs, like physician salaries, psychological services, NPs, or specialized tests)

Yearly increases are then determined based on a federal index for skilled nursing facilities, known as the Market-Basket Index. See below for further information on the PPS system and the legislative history.[45]

The facility bills for individual patients based on information supplied on the MDS. An example of the PPS for a Medicare Part A patient would be as follows:

Once the patient is admitted into the facility, MDS books are completed according to the following schedule counted from the initial day of admission: days five, fourteen, thirty, sixty, and ninety.

The patient is categorized on the MDS according to the RUG level into which he or she is classified. The classification is based on several factors pertaining to the patient: the

---

45 "Skilled Nursing Facility (SNF) Prospective Payment System, PPS Legislative History," Centers for Medicare & Medicaid Services, last modified July 31, 2013, accessed November 2016, https://www.cms.gov/Medicare/Medicare-Fee-for-Service-Payment/SNFPPS/Downloads/Legislative_History_07302013.pdf.

complexity of the clinical condition, special care requirements, decreased cognitive ability, limitations in physical function, and the amount of rehabilitation services (therapy) required. Performance on ADLs is also heavily weighted in the score. The facility's reimbursement increases with the increase of services provided, which ultimately achieves a higher RUG score.

Most facilities ensure that physical and occupational therapy evaluations are completed as soon as possible on the day of admission in order to begin treatment immediately to capture the maximum reimbursement. The prevailing point of view is that every patient will require at least these two therapy services. MDS books are completed with a projected number of minutes for therapy services. The applicable Medicare payment days for each of the completed MDS books is as follows:

ASSESSMENT TYPE	APPLICABLE MEDICARE PAYMENT DAYS*
5-Day	Days 1 through 14
14-Day	Days 15 through 30
30-Day	Days 31 through 60
60-Day	Days 61 through 90
90-Day	Days 91 through 100

*There are specific reference dates when each book is required to be completed as well as grace days that may be applied as needed.

In the event the patient for some reason is unable to complete the projected minutes—as set forth in the fifth and fourteenth day MDS book—by the fifteenth day, a change of therapy (COT) should be completed and submitted, although there may be circumstances when variables can be applied to forestall completing the COT. As these variables are not always applicable, every effort is made to record the minutes for the patient.

Therapists are advised that every attempt to see the patient, even if the patient is not feeling well and cannot fully participate in the scheduled therapy, is recorded as minutes spent. The minutes completed, along with other aforementioned areas, correspond to the RUG category, and that category carries with it a reimbursement amount. In the event the therapy minutes drop below the projected minutes for that period, the facility's reimbursement drops to the lower level. Thus, every effort is made to maintain the patient at the highest possible RUG level in order to avoid the facility having to revert to a lower reimbursement category.

In 2014, the House of Representatives passed a bill known as the *Improving Medicare Post-Acute Care Transformation Act* (also known as IMPACT Act of 2014)[46] for the purpose of tracking and improving Post-Acute care for Medicare beneficiaries. As a direct result, CMS developed the Continuity Assessment Record and Evaluation (or CARE) Item set which measures the health and functional status of Medicare beneficiaries upon discharge from acute care settings. As of October 2016, skilled-nursing facilities were required to submit functional and quality

---

46 *"Improving Medicare Post-Acute Care Transformation Act"*- IMPACT Act of 2014 H.R. 4994 113th Congress (2013-2014) accessed October 2017 Congress.gov https://www.congress.gov/bill/113th-congress/house-bill/4994

information in the form of patient assessments. The data for this information was to be collected from revisions MDS in sections A and a newly added section GG. Section GG (Functional Abilities and Goals) will be completed with each initial 5 day MDS PPS assessment as well as upon discharge. The person conducting the assessment scores the individual's usual performance for each activity using a 6-point scale as set forth with the CARE tool. This 6-point system differs significantly from the regular MDS 3.0 section G (ADLs). In the event the activity was not attempted at all, it is incumbent upon the person completing the assessment to indicate the reason it was not completed: patient refusal, medical or safety concerns or conditions or it was entirely not applicable.

Interestingly enough, as reported by Bloomberg News, the draft summary of the bill also required both the Medicare Payment Advisory Committee and CMS to issue reports to Congress by 2022 on ideas for new payment systems.[47]

CMS Recalibrates Rates

In May 2008 the CMS proposed recalibrating the reimbursement rates in order to prevent what it calculated to be a projected overpayment of $700 million.[48] In August 2008 it published the

---

47 N. Weixel *"Lawmakers Unveil Draft Legislation to Reform Post-Acute Care Payments"* Bloomberg BNA March 19, 2014 accessed October 2017 https://www.bna.com/law makers-unveil-draft-n17179885866/

48 73 Federal Register 25918, at 25923, May 7, 2008, accessed August 2017, http://frwebgate2.access.gpo.gov/cgi-bin/PDFgate.cgi?WAISdocID=FAFj8E/0/2/0&WAISact ion=retrieve.

final rates for skilled nursing facilities for the fiscal year ending 2009 and found that the overpayment had actually increased to $780.[49] The inspector general found that between 2006 and 2008 skilled nursing facilities had billed for higher-paying RUG categories, even though the characteristics of those receiving services were for the most part unchanged.[50]

The commission that advises Congress on Medicare policy, known as MedPAC (an acronym for Medicare Payment Advisory Commission), reviewed profit margins and operations for skilled nursing facilities and recommended in March 2008 that they receive no updates for the fiscal year 2009.[51] However, the CMS rejected that recommendation and gave the facilities an increase of 3.1 percent in the "market basket," which is an annual adjustment that accounts for cost of living and inflation. The result is an overpayment for fiscal year 2009 in the amount of a whopping $1.5 billion. According to commission's report to Congress, "CMS explicitly acknowledged that the nursing-home industry's intense lobbying campaign to prevent recalibration had been successful."[52]

The report goes on to state, "[I]n view of the widespread industry concern that a recalibration could potentially have

---

49 73 Federal Register 46416, at 46422, August 8, 2008, accessed August 2017, http://frwebgate1.access.gpo.gov/cgi-bin/PDFgate.cgi?WAISdocID=HcQhNJ/0/2/0&WAISaction=retrieve.

50 "Questionable Billing by Skilled Nursing Facilities," Office of Inspector General, accessed August 2017, http://oig.hhs.gov/oei/reports/oei-02-09-00202.pdf.

51 "Medicare Payment Policy, Report to Congress," The Medicare Payment Advisory Commission, accessed May 2017, www.medpac.gov/docs/default-source/reports/Mar08_EntireReport.pdf

52 "Medicare Reimbursement for Skilled Nursing Facilities Remains High"

adverse effects on beneficiaries and SNF clinical staff, and could negatively affect the quality of SNF care, we believe that the most prudent course is to continue to evaluate these issues carefully before proceeding."[53] The counter intuitiveness of this argument is staggering.

Given the concern that nursing-home patients and residents, clinical staff, and care provided would suffer if reimbursement rates were adjusted to avoid overpayment in billions of dollars, further stressing the economy and adding to an already-staggering deficit, the conclusion was to reward ownership with continued overpayment. The result, I'm sorry to say, is that through continued proliferation of corporate ownership, the care, staffing, and overall effect on recipients has continued to decline.

The CMA reported that the government was aware of overpayments to skilled nursing facilities since January 2006 and proposed a correction on a prospective basis. The irony to the situation is that CMA had concerns about the possible negative consequences it would have, most likely on the care that would be provided. Therefore, it concluded that going back to recover the excess payments made to SNFs since January 2006 would not be the most prudent means of proceeding. As an alternative, it decided to limit the scope for adjusting the rates to restoring the intended SNF PPS payments levels on a prospective basis only, effective October 1, 2010. One can only imagine the "negative consequences" it attempted to forestall that by all observation seem to have occurred despite the intention.

---

53 "Medicare Reimbursement for Skilled Nursing Facilities Remains High."

On April 27, 2017 CMS issued an advance notice for proposed changes for Medicare PPS reimbursement for SNFs to revise case-mix methodology. These changes are the result of evidence based literature and research by CMS and other entities regarding overcharges and manipulation of RUGs categories for financial gain. These proposed changes replace the use of RUGS categories with an entirely new classification system known as the Resident Classification System (RCS) which utilizes resident characteristics in determining reimbursement rather than services provided. The RCS would take into account five primary categories: major joint replacement, spinal surgery, other orthopedic, non-orthopedic surgery, acute neurologic, and medical management. These classifications seem to have roots in research that was conducted and considered as the basis for the bundled payment system. (Pertinent information on the bundled payment system is covered in the chapter by that name: Bundled-Payment System: An Alternative Reimbursement Method.) The proposed changes also separate payment for nursing and non-therapy services; combines payments for physical and occupational therapy but separates payment for speech/language pathology. Included are reductions for the per diem rate as the length of stay in the facility increases.[54]

You can view the Advance Notice of Proposed Rule Making at:

---

54 B.Ellsworth "The Beginning of the End of RUGs As We Know It" Health Dimensions Group April 28, 2017 accessed November 2017, http://healthdimensionsgroup.com/beginning-end-rugs-know/

https://s3.amazonaws.com/public-inspection.federalregister.gov/2017-08519.pdf

To date it is unclear when, in what manner, and if any of these proposed changes will take effect, especially as they will have a major impact on reimbursement for providers. Providers depend on maximizing RUG categories and lengths of stay as the foundation of their financial strategy. From my personal experience, as well as the experience of my colleagues, each system that has been developed and applied has found those at the top finding a way to apply, manipulate and find the loopholes in it for maximum gain; usually at the expense of both the beneficiaries and the professionals who provide care.

Concomitant with the aforementioned, CMS also proposed new potential measures to the Quality Reporting Program (QRP) and more specificity to the Value-Based Purchasing (VBP) program which addresses penalties for hospital readmissions. In addition, as of Fiscal Year 2020 reporting patient information become standardized according to 5 specific patient assessment categories required by law that include:

1. Functional status
2. Cognitive function
3. Special services, treatment and interventions
4. Medical conditions and co-morbidities, and
5. Impairments

Transitioning from Short-Term Rehabilitation to Long-Term Stay

• • •

Abuse and Neglect

It was an extremely hot summer day, and a resident was taken outside in the morning for sun. The resident was left outside in the sun through lunch and dinner; apparently no one knew the whereabouts of this person. When the resident was finally found, the resident was severely burned and was immediately taken to the hospital. Of course, the family called the state to report the incident, and family members of other residents also transferred their loved ones out of the facility. A similar incident occurred at a skilled-nursing facility in Florida.[55]

Therapy Minutes at all Costs

I was called to evaluate M. P., who was eating regular food when she was admitted. Almost overnight her condition had worsened to the point where she was so weak that she could not swallow solid foods or liquids.

After trying a few different feeding techniques with the patient and changing diet consistencies to those that might be easier to swallow, I was able to help her take in some food and liquid. I called the nurse and CNAs, instructed them in utilizing the appropriate feeding techniques, and recommended a downgrade in diet consistency to pureed solids while continuing with regular liquids.

I also recommended dysphagia therapy to improve the patient's swallowing abilities as well as making a recommendation to work with additional staff members on feeding techniques.

However, the following morning when I returned to the facility, M. P.'s condition had worsened even further. She was barely responsive and was no longer able to keep any solid food or liquid in her mouth. I immediately called the doctor to see the patient. We agreed that the best course of action on this Friday

---

55 "Man in Wheelchair, Left in the Sun at Florida Nursing Home, Dies," Fox News Health, accessed October 2016, http://www.foxnews.com/health/2016/05/03/man-in-wheelchair-left-in-sun-at-florida-nursing-home-dies.html.

morning was to hold off on trying to feed the patient for twenty-four hours, as her condition placed her at serious risk for aspiration, and to provide intravenous (IV) fluids. The doctor indicated that he was on call over the weekend and would determine how to proceed based on the patient's status the following day.

When I arrived at the facility Monday morning, my first order of business was to visit the patient. Her condition seemed further deteriorated. The doctor was already in the facility and informed me that the IV fluids had not had any positive effect on the patient's condition. On Saturday, with the family present, he had placed a small amount of food in the patient's mouth, but she was not able to tolerate it. After much deliberation, and based on the patient's expressed wishes prior to becoming ill, the decision was made to eliminate all IV fluids, maintain the order to discontinue feeding by mouth, and order a consultation for hospice care.

Further dysphagia therapy was obviously no longer warranted. I discharged the patient from the program and informed the director of the rehabilitation department.

However, later that day I saw the occupational therapist, who told me she was going to see the patient. "To do what?" I asked. She told me M. P. was still on the occupational-therapy program and that she had seen her in the morning and was seeing her again in the evening to move her around in bed. She said

M. P. was a Medicare patient, and she would continue seeing her for therapy until she was picked up by hospice. (Because hospice is considered end-of-life care, only under very specific and strict circumstances and only with prior approval can a patient receive any rehabilitation services.) She said there was no reason for her to just lie in bed in one position all day. I agreed, but I questioned whether that warranted a skilled rehabilitation service.

Part of the routine responsibility of the CNA who cares for patients is to provide range of motion and turn them in bed if they are unable to do so themselves. This patient was now barely responsive and apparently nearing the end of her *life,. I told the therapist I informed the director in the morning that the woman was clearly no longer a candidate for therapy, and I had taken her off the program. The therapist told me that the rehabilitation department director wanted her to continue seeing the patient.*

Clearly the purpose of continuing occupational therapy for this patient was only for the purpose of billing Medicare: maintaining a skilled-therapy service, which—along with the IV fluids—would qualify her for a higher facility reimbursement category. Was this in the patient's best interest? Had the family been made aware or informed of the decision? Would the family members want their mother to be used for money-making purposes? If the patient would not be considered a candidate for rehabilitation therapy once hospice care began, which in this case was the very next day, should the patient continue to be seen for therapy? The ethics of the decision to continue therapy services for this patient, and many others in similar circumstances, warrant serious consideration.

Therapy Minutes versus Outside Recreation or Family Excursions

I was recently seated in an area where the new director of the rehabilitation department was being trained and instructed in tracking and calculating therapy minutes for achieving the highest RUG categories. The regional director for the company, who was conducting the training, explained that if the patient, specifically the Medicare patient, was nearing the end of the time period in which the minutes were being counted for the highest category and missed a therapy day because he or she was sick or had a medical appointment outside of the facility, any other outside excursions should be discouraged in order to maintain that ultrahigh-RUG category (this included outings with family or any other nonessential excursions).

• • •

THOUGH OFTEN UNANTICIPATED AND CERTAINLY unwanted, there are circumstances that result in a patient being unable to return home after the completion of a stay on a short-term rehabilitation unit. The transition can be difficult for both the patient and family and/or caregivers who have bonded with particular staff members or developed friendships with other patients on the rehabilitation unit. Ultimately this can create a sense of loss. There are several factors that may contribute to the need to transition from the short-term-care unit to the long-term-care unit.

One factor is that the patient has not made sufficient progress to return home, and, depending on the type of insurance, continuation of payment for therapy services is denied. Insurance reimbursement is usually based on the patient's progress toward meeting the goals, as set forth during the initial evaluation. There may be a variety of reasons for the reduced progress: overall weakness or frailty, complicated medical status, nature or extent of the impairment or deficits, or inability to participate in exercise or therapy to the necessary extent. There are also circumstances when—despite repeated efforts—the patient is just not able to respond to the treatment provided.

Other circumstances that may preclude the patient from returning home may be a home situation that is not conducive to meet the patient's continued or extended medical, physical, or cognitive needs. There may be difficult access, like steps, that the patient with persisting physical impairment may not be able to negotiate. There may also be barriers within the home that interfere with ease of movement, either with a wheelchair or a walker. Insufficient family support or reimbursement for the necessary community services to provide adequate support for a safe discharge may be another factor impacting the move from short-term rehabilitation. (If a family member requires long-term home care, this is not a Medicare-reimbursable expense.) Therefore, there are alternative financial arrangements that will need to be made.

Medicare and most private insurance companies do not pay for a long-term-care stay, which means if long-term-care insurance is not already in place, the family may need to apply for Medicaid. The social worker on the rehabilitation unit should be helpful in providing assistance for completing the paperwork in this process. Approval takes time—in most cases at least several weeks and in some cases months. However, the patient goes into Medicaid-pending status during this process.

It should be noted that placement on a long-term-care unit does not necessarily mean that the person will never return home. I have personally seen situations where the most unlikely patients, even ones with severe physical or medical impairments and deteriorated cognitive conditions, return home with significant family and community support services. However, this requires extensive strategic planning and cooperation between the facility and family, which may take a protracted period of time. Thus, the person will remain on the long-term-care unit until all the details are arranged.

Families and caregivers are informed about a patient's inability to return home in a meeting with a social worker or as part of a care-plan meeting. The reality of the move from short-term rehabilitation to the long-term-care unit is understandably a very emotionally charged situation for both the patient and the family. There may be anger, disappointment, blame, guilt, and depression, and both the patient and family should seek help in dealing with these feelings.

If long-term care is needed, the patient will most likely be transferred to a long-term-care unit in the rehabilitation facility; in some circumstances, the patient may need to be transferred to an entirely different facility. Either way there are situations of which both the patient and the family or caregivers should be aware.

First and foremost, the status changes from that of patient to that of a resident, because the facility is considered the person's new home. This is more than a term of verbiage; there are significant connotations that go along with this change.

In most facilities, the long-term-care unit has a very different appearance and feel than that of the short-term-rehabilitation unit. The extra care, resident attention, and philosophy of customer service are not as pronounced. In many facilities, especially those that have been redesigned to capture the appearance of the chandelier effect, the surroundings of the short-term rehabilitation unit are top notch, even plush; ownership stops at nothing to satisfy the needs and desires of the patients and their families and makes the surroundings as beautiful as possible. It is suggested that families visit the long-term unit of the facility to determine if the discrepancy in appearance and services is too great. Talk to families of other residents and the local ombudsman regarding questions or concerns about the unit and quality of care.

In some cases, the nursing home with the rehabilitation unit is not geographically conducive to where family members reside. In that case the social worker would recommend facilities in closer proximity to the family members' residences to allow for ease of visitation. The social worker would help determine the facilities that have bed availability and can meet the patient's potential medical and rehabilitation needs. Families and caregivers should visit those facilities as well and ask as many questions as possible to determine if it is a suitable situation for their loved one as well as to determine insurance acceptance, coverage, and any out-of-pocket expenses.

There are groups one can contact for questions or guidance. (See the appendix for a list of agencies and/or groups to contact for information.)

Many residents on long-term-care units are sicker, frailer, and more debilitated, often with varying stages of dementia, which admittedly can be very upsetting. Try to find the unit in the facility that would be most suitable for your loved one. Oftentimes units are chosen based on bed availability. Work closely with the social worker, and be a strong advocate so that your loved one does not find himself or herself on a unit that will add to the feelings he or she may already have about moving to a long-term-care situation.

If your loved one does not speak the predominant language of most of the facility staff members, inquire if there are staff members who speak the language and, if so, the shifts they are on duty so that your loved one does not feel isolated or unable to convey needs, wants, or feelings. Some facilities develop a language database of sorts that lists staff members, the shifts they work, and the languages they speak.

One would intuitively think that admissions coordinators would be aware of this information and be up-front about whether or not they can meet a patient's needs when considering an individual for admission who does not speak the predominant language of most of the workers in the facility. Unfortunately, in all the facilities I have worked, I have rarely known this to be the case. Therefore, it will be incumbent upon the family member or loved one to be assertive about developing a means for the staff to communicate with the resident.

Alternatively, one could speak with the speech/language pathologist about developing a communication board or other means by which the resident could communicate with staff and vice versa. There are cell phone and iPad applications that may be used for translation. Phone interpreter services, like www.languageline.com, provide on-demand, phone-interpreter services twenty-four hours a day, seven days a week, for 365 days a year. The company has nearly nine thousand professional interpreters who fluently speak over 240 languages. However, this process can be cumbersome, especially if staff are attending to a resident in a room some distance away from a phone. In addition, there are often staff shortages and time constraints that render this process awkward.

Long-term-care units often do not have the same number of activities or opportunities for stimulation. The pace can be slower, and there may be fewer staff members available to meet residents' needs. You may want to speak with the director of recreation or the activity staff member assigned to the unit regarding any special interests or hobbies the resident may have. Transitions to a long-term stay often evoke feelings of isolation, loneliness, anger, and depression. Engaging residents with activities provides a means for them to connect with others as well as to keep as physically and mentally active as possible.

Upon arriving on the long-term-care unit, the resident will be greeted by either the nurse manager of the unit or the nurse assigned to him or her. Oftentimes it will be that person, a nursing assistant, or another staff member who will show the new resident around the unit and orient him or her to the new surroundings. Usually there are other new staff members to meet who are associated with the long-term-care unit. The resident may have a different doctor or NP, as well as a different social worker, dietitian, and activities or recreation therapist.

Medical records transfer from one unit to another within a facility. However, the new staff members may conduct their own new assessments and generate new reports regarding the resident's needs on that unit.

Daily routines may be conducted at different times. Meal times, laundry pick-up and delivery, and shower or bath schedule days all may be slightly different. Rehabilitation services—physical, occupational, and speech therapy—can continue on the long-term-care unit if needed, but frequency and duration may change.

Even though schedules may change, families should advocate for their loved one. Feel free to inform the staff about your loved one's bathing needs and preferences; they are obligated to meet those needs as closely as possible, regardless of the facility's staffing issues.

THE ROOM AS THE NEW HOME

Though some short-term units have single-bed rooms, many have double-occupancy rooms. When moving to a long-term-care unit, having a roommate may not be a significant change. What may be different, however, is that on the short-term unit, many patients spend most of the day out of their rooms in therapy. On the long-term-care unit, this may not be the case.

There are instances where roommates do not get along because of personality differences, degree of medical or cognitive issues, or personal preferences (e.g., early or late rising or bed times, TV times or loudness levels, room temperature preferences). If these issues cannot be resolved, discuss a room change with the staff and/or social worker.

In order for the new surroundings to feel more like home, some facilities will allow the resident's family to bring a favorite chair, bookcase, or other furniture item from home if the room is large enough. Family members may also bring special throw pillows, blankets, lamps, decorations, or bedspreads, as well as favorite music, books, personal mementos, and pictures. Favorite newspapers or magazines can be delivered to the resident, albeit at an additional charge, if you or other friends or family members are not able to personally bring them to the facility.

Some facilities have private rooms or areas where families and friends can share visits or even special meals. Make sure you inquire about any special dietary or food-consistency restrictions that the physician has ordered for the resident based on his or her particular medical or physical condition. In the event you disagree with the foods or food consistencies that have been ordered, make sure you request appropriate meetings or evaluations with the unit nurse manager, dietitian, speech pathologist, and/or doctor to review those issues. It is a serious matter to give a resident food that is not allowed and can result in serious medical or health complications.

Some units have a TV in every room, while others may have a central TV on the unit. You may be allowed to bring the resident's TV from home or a smaller desktop unit. TVs and radios with headphones are ideal, so the resident can use them without disturbing roommates.

Telephones may be installed in the room at an additional charge; inquire about the cost before the resident arrives on the unit so that appropriate plans can be made. Many residents feel isolated if they don't have a way of contacting their families, especially in the initial time after moving to the long-term-care unit. Nowadays many residents who are capable prefer using a cell phone, but cell phones can also be easily lost or misplaced.

All nursing homes have an event calendar that is posted in the residents' rooms, but this monthly calendar of events is often difficult to read. Announcements are usually made on an overhead sound system to alert residents of significant upcoming activities, like movies, music programs, and religious services. However, depending on your loved one's status (cognitive, hearing, vision), he or she may not be able to hear the announcements or read the calendars. Though a representative from the activities department will visit the resident to find out likes, dislikes, and preferences, it would be a good idea for you to share this information with that staff member. If the recreation therapist is aware of a particular interest, he or she will visit the resident and encourage attendance at a particular activity or event when it occurs.

Not all facilities are wired for Wi-Fi, though an increasing number are since access to the Internet is important to so many in this day and age. If a computer is important to your loved one, some facilities have a central area where computers are available for residents to use. If not, inquire about use of a laptop if this is appropriate.

AFTER THE MOVE

It is ideal to be with your loved one at the time of the move to the long-term-care unit, although this is not always possible. However, it is of the utmost importance that you get to know the staff on the unit where your loved one is now a resident. Though they will receive pertinent information from the short-term unit, staff members will appreciate your input regarding the resident's likes and dislikes, preferences, and even behavior as you know it.

Remember that you are your loved one's advocate, and do not hesitate to speak up to the appropriate parties regarding issues or concerns. Oftentimes people feel there will be repercussions if they complain or speak up about concerning issues; *this should never happen.* In the unfortunate circumstance where negative consequences occur, there are channels to take the matter further. If need be, disciplinary actions will be taken. There is an expression—the squeaky wheel gets the oil. It also applies to this setting. If it is known that family members and loved ones are involved or watching, it goes a long way in keeping staff on their toes.

Participate in all care-plan meetings. If you are not able to personally attend, phone conferences can be set up at a convenient time for all parties concerned. The care-plan meeting is one in which all aspects of the resident's needs are discussed and planned: medical condition, rehabilitation, nursing, dietary, activities, and more. A full care plan is devised once per year and upon any significant changes the resident may experience. Updates to the care plan are made on a quarterly basis—every three months. Residents and their loved ones should always be informed and invited to these meetings.

Facilities are required to have family council meetings. Attend those as frequently as you can to keep abreast of issues within the facility that will impact your loved one. Visit as often as possible and at different times of the day, including weekends if possible. This will give you a good feel for how the facility and staff function at different times.

If your loved one is able, visits outside the facility can be arranged. They must be approved by the resident's facility doctor and deemed safe by the nursing and rehabilitation staff. Oftentimes facilities do not authorize outside visits in the first thirty days in order to fully assess the resident's functioning and overall capability.

ADDITIONAL CONSIDERATIONS

There may be additional paperwork to complete if the resident is going to a long-term-care unit at another facility. In the event you have already addressed these issues, this is not new information. If you have not addressed these issues, discussing topics like advance directives may be upsetting. When an individual has made advance arrangements in the event he or she becomes incapable of making decisions regarding personal care, that person has appointed a designated party to make decisions on the individual's behalf through what is known as a durable power of attorney for health care or a health-care proxy. This is one type of advance directive.

A second type of advance directive is known as a living will or health-care declaration. In this type of directive, an individual has set forth exactly what type of care he or she would be willing, or not willing, to accept in an end-of-life decision. If the resident is not sufficiently alert and has not already made his or her wishes known in these areas by means of the living will or health-care declaration, these decisions will be the responsibility of a person who has been designated to sign the appropriate papers. Oftentimes this involves difficult decisions about how much treatment to provide and for how long, and these situations can be rife with family disagreement.

* *Advance directives* include information related to resuscitation and other forms of care that would preserve life with artificial sustaining measures. Among those are cardiopulmonary resuscitation (CPR, which is the emergency restarting of the person's heart), use of a ventilator (a

machine that essentially breathes for the person), dialysis (a machine that provides kidney function when the body's kidneys have failed), tube or IV feeding (when the person can no longer safely eat or swallow), and antibiotics (to fight or stave off a life-threatening infection).

- A *Do Not Resuscitate directive (DNR)* indicates that, in the event of a medical emergency, no measures will be used to resuscitate the resident—essentially allowing nature to take its course. This could result in the resident dying. There are some states in which this is referred to as Physician's Order for Life-Sustaining Treatment (POLST).

- There are also *Do Not Hospitalize directives (DNH)* and *Do Not Intubate directives (DNI)*, which are usually discussed when and if the resident's physical, medical, and/or mental status has deteriorated to the point where the inevitable end of life appears to be approaching. A person's age may be an additional factor that is considered when making these decisions.

Other levels of care that may be considered are *palliative care* or *hospice care.*

- *Palliative care* is a specialty that focuses on relieving symptoms of pain and stress associated with serious illness, regardless of the diagnosis. Though it is often associated with end-of-life care, it can occur at any stage of an illness, and it generally means that the measures applied are intended to keep the patient comfortable, thus the name *comfort care*. However, palliative care can do more than merely keep a resident comfortable. Palliative or comfort-care measures do not preclude other forms of restorative or aggressive treatments. All other treatments can still be in place if palliative care is applied.

- *Hospice care* is a subcategory under palliative care and is considered end-of-life care, which means that no additional treatment or curative measures will be pursued. When considering hospice care, a special hospice nurse from an outside agency will be assigned to the resident. In the facilities in which I have worked, the hospice nurse is from an agency that has a contractual agreement with that facility. The hospice nurse will visit and evaluate the patient, taking into consideration all aspects of the condition and ultimately making a decision as to whether the patient will be accepted into the hospice-care program. In the event the patient is accepted, the patient will receive individualized attention for a designated number of hours per day provided by the hospice-care agency. Enrolling in hospice is not necessarily the end of life. There have been many instances, which I have personally witnessed, where the patient improved considerably and was then discharged from hospice. At any time the family or the individual can request discharge from hospice.

Conversations about a long-term stay in a facility may be difficult for all family members. For assistance, you may visit CareConversations.org.

MDS: Minimum Data Set 3.0

• • •

Minimum Data Set (MDS) is a reporting system mandated by the federal government. MDS reports the conditions of all individuals, regardless of their payment source, in all facilities certified to accept Medicare or Medicaid reimbursement. In most cases it is coordinated and/or completed by a registered nurse who must meet specific requirements in order to be certified in MDS completion. Other professionals may contribute to the completion of the MDS; the finished process must be signed off by the registered nurse. At the time of this writing, MDS Version 3.0 is used for those enrolled in Medicare and Medicaid and beneficiaries of all other insurances.

Prior to 2006 the MDS was used merely as a means for the department of health in each state to track the conditions of residents and the concomitant care they required within a facility. The MDS was completed at specific intervals, upon admission and then on a quarterly basis throughout the year. Following this pattern an MDS book, as it is known, was completed for each resident on an annual basis. Subsequently a shortened-version book was completed on a quarterly basis for each year that the individual resided in the facility. Once completed the information on the MDS was electronically transmitted to an MDS database in that particular state; that information was then captured in a national MDS database at the CMS.

However, in 2006 the previous system that was in use for calculating payment to facilities (the Peer Review Instrument [PRI] in New York State) was deemed insufficient for reporting on patient information for purposes of determining reimbursement. Since the MDS was a more comprehensive review of an individual's condition and the care required to meet patient needs (e.g., medical, psychosocial, behavioral, or rehabilitative), the MDS became the system to drive all reimbursement for Medicare- and Medicaid-approved nursing homes and skilled nursing facilities.

While the same MDS book is completed for both Medicare and Medicaid recipients, there are slight differences in the intervals for completion as well as the information that is obtained from those books and how the books are used. The facility is paid on a PPS for Medicare Part A beneficiaries, and the interval for book completion is based on the projected rehabilitation or other special services delivered to the patient, based on an initial assessment. The MDS book is completed at prescribed intervals for Medicare recipients as follows: five days, fourteen days, thirty days, sixty days, and ninety days.

The ninety-day book is the last PPS book completed before the one hundred Medicare days near completion. The RUG scores that are calculated for Medicare recipients under this PPS system, based on therapy minutes, vary slightly from the RUG score minutes once the individual transitions out of Medicare. If at any time the individual does not maintain the levels of therapy services that have been projected, the facility—absent changes in the book completion date—completes a Change of Therapy MDS book, and the reimbursement rate slides back to the category that corresponds to the new RUG score. Every effort is made to avoid this situation.

Whether the individual transitions out of Medicare to Medicaid or any other insurance or is admitted to the facility with those type of insurances as a long-term-care resident, an OBRA MDS book is completed. The name is taken from OBRA '87, upon which the principles of the book are based. These MDS books are completed according to a different schedule. There is an initial, comprehensive-assessment MDS book completed upon admission, and abbreviated books are completed quarterly (approximately every ninety days) until another annual comprehensive book is completed at the anniversary of the initial book. This schedule continues unless there is a significant change in the resident, at which point a comprehensive, significant-change MDS book is completed. The cycle continues from that point forward.

This entire cycle continues until an MDS discharge book is completed in the event the resident is discharged from the facility. It should be noted that every resident will have at least two MDS books throughout the year that fall during the Case-Mix Index (CMI) process. As discussed in the chapter on CMI, when those books are due it is incumbent upon the staff within the facility to examine each resident closely in order to maximize the RUG scores for the books, which thereby maximizes reimbursement.

If a regular quarterly MDS book is completed during the CMI period, but it is noted that a significant change in the resident has occurred, warranting additional services that can be captured to increase the RUG category (e.g., rehabilitation, special treatments), then an additional significant-change book will be completed at that time as well. In most cases every effort is made to coordinate additional treatments with the scheduled

MDS book, as there are specific requirements that must be met before a significant-change MDS book can be completed.

The first area (Section A) which is completed on the comprehensive MDS Version 3.0 includes pertinent identifying information. The following is a list of the areas that are scored:

1. Section B - Hearing, Speech, and Vision
2. Section C - Cognitive Patterns
3. Section D - Mood
4. Section E - Behavior
5. Section F – Preferences for Customary Routine and Activities
6. Section G – Functional Status
7. Section H – Bladder and Bowel
8. Section I – Active Disease Diagnosis
9. Section J – Health Conditions
10. Section K – Swallowing and Nutritional Status
11. Section L – Oral/Dental Status
12. Section M – Skin Conditions
13. Section O – Special Treatments and Procedures
14. Section P - Restraints
15. Section Q – Participation in Assessment and Goal Setting
16. Section T - Therapy supplement for PPS.

While the MDS is the instrument that is the driving force for facility reimbursement, it does not stand alone as a comprehensive assessment of the individual within the facility for the OBRA Medicaid assessment. Rather the MDS is one part of the

Resident Assessment Instrument (RAI) and plays a major role in identifying actual or potential areas of concern that will lead to the necessary planning for interventions to meet the resident's needs within the facility. The other areas contributing to the resident assessment are the Care Area Assessments (or CAAs) and the Comprehensive Care Plan (CCP).

The CAAs are completed for the initial (admission) MDS book and upon annual review, significant change in status, or significant correction of a prior full assessment and provide a more in-depth identification of areas of concern for a particular resident. The CAAs must also be completed when a Medicare assessment is combined with a comprehensive clinical assessment (as when the patient completes a Medicare Part A stay and remains in the facility under a different insurance source). Once these areas are identified or triggered, as they are colloquially known, they become care area triggers (CATs). CATs may necessitate further evaluation and would result in more involvement from the interdisciplinary team (IDT) to investigate the causes and contributing factors for these triggered areas.

Once evaluations for a resident are completed, a more in-depth intervention plan is undertaken and becomes the framework upon which the CCP is developed. It is important to note that though each triggered CAA requires an assessment, those areas may or may not be found to warrant a care-plan intervention. If the condition is found to be a sufficient problem to warrant an intervention on the care plan, the IDT must take into consideration whether the intervention will serve to eliminate, reverse, or maintain the current level of function and avoid further deterioration.

It is important to note that there are no mandates under the federal guidelines for how a nursing home or skilled-nursing facility uses these CAAs in addressing areas of concern and developing appropriate interventions. That becomes a subjective process within each facility, based on the staff, the resources available, and the creativity with which the staff can address the residents' needs.

The assessment of care areas on the MDS 3.0 are as follows:

1. Delirium
2. Cognitive Loss/Dementia
3. Visual Function
4. Communication
5. ADL Functional/Rehabilitation Potential
6. Urinary Incontinence and Indwelling Catheter
7. Psychosocial Well-Being
8. Mood State
9. Behavioral Symptoms
10. Activities
11. Falls
12. Nutritional Status
13. Feeding Tubes
14. Dehydration/Fluid Maintenance
15. Dental Care
16. Pressure Ulcer
17. Psychotropic Medication Use
18. 18. Physical Restraints
19. Pain
20. Return to Community Referral

The information obtained on the CAA serves to assist the IDT in the following ways.

1. Identify associated causes and effects that may contribute to the condition (e.g., is a fall related to a medication change, change in mental status, equipment failure, staffing issue?).
2. Are multiple triggered conditions related to each other?
3. Is there sufficient reason to investigate the reason for the condition from family members, assigned guardians, prior residence, doctors, and caregivers on the unit on varying shifts?
4. Will rehabilitation intervention address the condition, and is the resident a candidate?
5. Should specialized laboratory or diagnostic tests be ordered? (in-house or outside of the facility)
6. Does the condition warrant referral to an outside specialist (e.g., neurology) or a specialty within the facility? (e.g., psychology)
7. Formulate care plan goals, strategies, and interventions.

According to Chapter 4 of CMS's "Resident Assessment Instrument Version 3.0 User's Manual," the documentation that addresses each triggered CAA should include the following:

1. The nature of the issue or condition (may or may not include objective data, as well as subjective complaints)
2. Causes and contributing factors

3. Complications affecting or caused by the particular care area for the resident
4. Risk factors resulting from the condition that affect the staff's decision to include it on the care plan
5. Considerations that would determine the interventions on the care plan. (i.e., including appropriate and necessary documentation to justify the decision to proceed or not to proceed with care planning)
6. The reason for the need for referrals to appropriate specialists for further evaluation, whether inside or outside of the facility
7. Identifying the appropriate research, resources(s), or assessment tool(s) that were used in performing the CAA. Only sources that are not considered standard sources used for this CAA by facility policy need be identified.
8. Completion of Section V (CAA Summary).[56]

Patients or residents and their families may obtain copies of the medical record, which may include a list of medications, evaluations, and the care plan at a cost per page. However, those same interested parties do not necessarily have access to the MDS, CAAs, or CATs.

It is this writer's contention that it would be in those parties' best interest to request and be able to receive those documents in order to ensure accuracy of reporting on the resident's

---

56 "Resident Assessment Instrument Version 3.0 User's Manual," Centers for Medicare & Medicaid Services, accessed January 2017 https://www cms.gov/Medicare/Quality-Initiatives.../MDS-30-RAI-Manual-V113.pdf.

condition to the state department of health and ultimately the CMS, as well as to validate that information isn't inaccurately scored in order to somehow receive reimbursement for a condition when its existence, or severity, is questionable.

Of special importance to families or loved ones of the resident is that upon completion of the initial comprehensive MDS and at subsequent completion of the annual MDS, there is a care-plan meeting to which family members must be invited. This invitation comes via phone and mail. The importance of family and/or loved one involvement cannot be stressed enough in ensuring that needed care is rendered properly and that medications are not rendered unnecessarily—as well as keeping abreast of accurate reporting of all information related to the resident. All care of the resident is nursing driven and must be accompanied and substantiated by nursing notes. One can always request nursing notes to ensure the reporting of situations and conditions as they pertain to the resident is completed in the most accurate fashion.

Not all facilities conduct care-plan meetings upon completion of the quarterly assessment, and if they do these meetings are often done in a more informal manner. Not all facilities conduct care-plan meetings for significant-change assessments and the completion of the MDS books. However, the family or loved one must be notified of any change pertaining to the resident, (e.g., medication, room change, change in condition, mood change). and there must be documentation of this notification in the resident's chart. In the event the family is notified that a significant change has occurred, it is within the family's rights to request an interdisciplinary meeting for the significant change and request any documentation attesting to the change.

There have been instances where documentation shows that families were notified when they were not. In some cases, these changes give the license to administer services and medications that may not be necessary but that will increase the resident's RUG score, thereby increasing facility reimbursement. This occurs because the relationship among department heads (e.g., rehabilitation directors, MDS coordinators, nursing, and social services) is such that it can create an environment where, because everyone is under pressure from administration and/or ownership to obtain the highest scores in an effort to maximize the reimbursement rate, information may sometimes be reported that is not necessarily accurate and is not in the best interest of the resident. Therefore, it is incumbent upon the family and/or loved one to be vigilant and be the resident's advocate, especially as cognitive status (e.g., dementia, Alzheimer's disease), age-related frailty, or illness which may preclude residents from being their own best advocates.

Active advocacy is unfortunately almost counterintuitive to the reasons and situations that result in nursing-home placement. Distance from family and families that are preoccupied with their own busy lives, as well as lack of interest in elders in their declining years, make advocacy more difficult. The thought that someone else will care for residents is far too easy and sometimes not fully accurate. The result is unnecessary or inadequate care for the sake of profit.

While there appears to be greater regulation by oversight agencies who review information concerning the resident's condition—especially ADLs, where there is a section introduced on the MDS aimed specifically at addressing functional status—there are situations where the nursing notes and MDS scores may coincide. However, this is not a true representation of the resident's status. I have personally seen such discrepancies on many occasions.

While the department of health or other oversight bodies may look at the documentation to ensure that the representation of the information is consistent and accurate, there is no way the bodies can examine the resident to ensure that the information is an accurate representation of the resident's actual condition or state of being and that this information is accurately reflected in the treatment or care being provided.

First, therapists who are being pressured to complete their work with increasing emphasis on high productivity may at times merely complete MDS sections based on previous assessments, without even viewing the resident. I have also known instances where MDS coordinators complete the assessment for the therapists. The best MDS coordinators visit the resident to see for themselves; many merely rely on reporting from nursing or other staff members.

Case-Mix Index: Use and Misuse

• • •

Inflating CMI Scores

My extremely caring and attentive friend was working as a nurse manager at a facility when a new director of rehabilitation arrived shortly after the facility was acquired by a for-profit corporation. As CMI period approached, the director of the rehabilitation department submitted a list of residents he wanted picked up for both occupational and physical therapy. Many of these residents had been in the facility for many years and now had limited alertness and responsiveness as well as long-standing contractures, many of them were also wheelchair bound and/or bedridden. They were dependent in all aspects of care. The director insisted the nurse write notes justifying the patient's candidacy for rehabilitation services.

Not only did she refuse, there were family members who were irate that their loved ones would be subjected to this type of intervention. They felt their loved ones were resting comfortably in their final stages of life and should not be disturbed. One family member in particular threatened to call the state if her mother was picked up for any type of therapy program.

After considerable pressure the nurse sarcastically suggested, "Maybe I should bring my houseplants, and you could try and rehabilitate them as well." She in no way meant that she was comparing the patients to houseplants. She is an extremely kind, caring, and attentive nurse. The outrage that sparked this statement was related to the fact that these were attempts to go to any means to heighten a CMI score; proof of misuse of the system for financial gain. The nurse manager went so far as to consult with the NP in the facility, questioning if what the director of rehabilitation was requesting was in fact legal. She was told that it was legal, although it was taking the spirit of the law to the very edge of what would be considered legal. The question was whether or not it was ethical.

Therapy for CMI Purposes—Misuse for Financial Gain

A registered occupational therapist told me of a facility in which she worked where the director of the rehabilitation department instructed her to see a patient with a minimal response level for sixty minutes. She attempted to reason with the director, informing him that the resident was not a candidate for that level of service, but he insisted—especially because it was the crucial CMI period. Though the therapist acquiesced for that patient, she told me she left shortly thereafter, as soon as she was able to secure work in another facility.

Rehabilitation and Profit

A director of rehabilitation with whom I worked was affiliated with a not-for-profit facility that was in the process of being bought by a well-known, corporate entity. The corporation asked her to stay on as director of the department. As part of her decision-making process, she went to a corporate meeting with other directors from that company. She told me the corporate rehabilitation director presented the company's expectations. A high percentage of Medicare patients must receive the maximum number of minutes (ultrahigh category), and at least 50 percent of the facility patients were to be picked up during CMI, resulting in an expected CMI score range. The director presented a list of other expectations, including productivity demands for therapists.

These items were nonnegotiable—no questions were to be asked, and the goals were to be achieved no matter what. My friend told me there was no talk of patient care, service delivery, quality of care, therapist experience, education, or incentives. It was all numbers and revenue driven. She said that as she sat in that meeting, she made her decision. She returned to the facility, where she had been a successful and appreciated rehabilitation director for a number of years, and submitted her letter of resignation.

Rehabilitation Need for CMI Purposes—The Wrong View

I was speaking to the director of the rehabilitation department and expressed concern that a new patient had an order for a swallow evaluation entered in the computer on September 24, but I was not told about it until October 2. The physician recommended the evaluation after receiving a report that the patient was coughing while drinking liquids.

The director's response was that it was particularly important to complete the evaluation because CMI was approaching. It was important to pick up as many people as possible. My concern was an entirely different matter. If the patient was experiencing swallowing difficulty while drinking, which could ultimately result in aspiration and compromise the patient's health and well-being, then I should have been informed of the situation immediately. The patient should not have been waiting for over a week. The director's concern was obviously entirely misplaced.

● ● ●

MEDICAID PATIENTS IN A LONG-TERM stay receive reimbursement for services from state public funding sources in many ways. One of the systems with the most widespread use across the country—approximately thirty-five states use this system—is the Case-Mix reimbursement system, which was designed to reimburse facilities based on the services they provide to residents as opposed to a calculation based purely on facility and low-volume costs.

The calculation for the CMI is based on a three-month period that occurs twice yearly. The beginning of CMI is calculated by the following formula: ninety-two days back from the last Wednesday in January. The same holds true for the CMI period that begins ninety-two days back from the last Wednesday in July. Under this system patients are picked up for therapeutic intervention for specific amounts of time over a specific period of time. These interventions are then reported to the state via the MDS for the purposes of determining the reimbursement rate for the facility.

Residents fall into particular categories based on the amount of rehabilitation therapy services they receive, as well as other medical and nursing interventions. The more extensive the services provided, the higher the reimbursement rate. The thinking behind this method is that if a facility is caring for residents who require more extensive or heavy care, it should receive funds concomitant with the resident's condition, the level of care provided for that condition, and associated expenditures related to that level.

Furthermore, it was felt that if facilities were reimbursed according to patient-care needs, they would be more likely to provide that care, and it could improve efficiency of payment. The rate is, therefore, based on services provided. As the system has been applied, there have been serious concerns raised that are worthy of consideration.

1. Facilities may be less likely to accept residents who would require lighter care because they will fall into a lower payment category; these patients could potentially encounter difficulty when seeking nursing-home placement.
2. As residents improve they will be reclassified into a lower payment category, and management may not look favorably on helping residents improve.
3. Facilities can increase profits by spending less than the rate that was calculated from the CMI score and may not provide the appropriate care to those patients once admitted—essentially withholding care and constituting negligence.
4. The framework for how decisions are made is financial in nature rather than based on resident need.

There are also incentives or add-ons that have been given to facilities as encouragement for accepting residents deemed to require considerably more care because of the nature or extent of their conditions and/or who otherwise may have had difficulty gaining nursing-home acceptance (e.g., ventilator-dependent patients, those with Alzheimer's or dementia, and those who are brain injured). Some states require additional programming or staffing to care for these residents, while others are given the additional funds merely for admitting these residents. This incentivizes accepting residents without having to spend money to care for them.

Other states offer this add-on rate for residents who require specialized equipment or expensive treatments due to their medical conditions. An example of an add-on or incentive that requires additional programming would be a facility that admits ventilator-dependent patients but must either submit an individualized care plan for each patient—which is then subject to independent review—or make program and staffing adjustments to meet those needs.

An example of the opposite scenario is one in which there is a rate adjustment for a facility accepting residents with moderate to severe cognitive impairment without a requirement for any specialized programming. It is this writer's contention that any facility that receives additional reimbursement for accepting patients or residents with a specialized condition *should be required* to allocate funds for improving the quality of care through additional staffing, staff training, and programmatic or environmental changes to address those needs.

The Long-Term Care Community Coalition (LTCCC) March 2009 report entitled "Modifying the Case-Mix Medicaid Nursing Home System to Encourage Quality, Access, and Efficiency,"[57] provides a list of add-ons and incentives by state and can be viewed at www.ltccc.org. To view more recent

---

57 R. Mollot and C. Rudder "Modifying the Case-Mix Medicaid Nursing Home System to Encourage Quality, Access and Efficiency" The Long Term Care Community Coalition Oct. 2009 accessed March 2017, http://theconsumervoice.org/uploads/files/events/Using-Medicaid-Reimbursement-System-Mollot-Rudder-PPT.pdf

information regarding your particular state's add-ons or incentives for nursing-home facilities, visit your state's website.

CMI Process in Practice

During the biannual, three-month periods that end the last Wednesday in January and the last Wednesday in July, long-term-care residents having straight Medicaid or Medicaid plus Medicare Part B coverage are examined closely for any therapy (occupational, physical, speech) that can be offered with the underlying premise of improving function or quality of care. Residents are also looked at to determine their candidacy for any other extensive services that can be applied and reported by the facility (e.g., IV therapy, as one example). The services that are delivered to a particular resident equate to a RUG level. Each RUG level is then assigned a numerical score or Case-Mix Index. At the end of the three-month period, the CMIs for Medicaid MDSs are averaged to obtain the facility's overall CMI score. That score equates to a dollar amount the facility will then receive as the daily reimbursement rate for Medicaid patients. This is based on the most recent OBRA MDS levels.

While instituting specific periods of time for facilities to examine their populations and report residents who require heavier care seems to be astute, it is actually a cumbersome and convoluted system that is highly manipulated for the specific purpose of increasing revenue. An August 2011 article by Christopher S. Brunt and John R. Bowblis focuses on Medicare reimbursement, and it is also applicable to the situation with the

CMI time period. The authors found that skilled nursing facilities increase therapy minutes and vary the thresholds to define Case Mix in order to achieve higher rates of reimbursement.[58]

During this period rehabilitation department directors, MDS coordinators, and nurses usually work in close cooperation to find residents within the facility who can be picked up for programming. These residents are selected based on their MDS book due dates, as services must be provided for five days within a seven-day period prior to the day the MDS is to be completed. The required date for MDS book completion is also known as the assessment reference date, commonly called the ARD date. The date selected for the completion of the MDS book should reflect the maximum number of services provided.

There is usually a feverish pitch in the attempt to capture as many residents for services as possible. Therapists have been known to be pressured to either pick up residents who are not clinically appropriate or to deliver the maximum number of minutes to residents—their protestations usually falling on deaf ears. I have also known of instances when, after providing service and recording the therapy time provided, therapists' minutes have been changed to reflect a higher RUG category. This also happens because rehabilitation department directors are under pressure from their superiors to achieve the highest scores possible.

---

58 J. R. Bowblis and C. S. Brunt, "Medicare Skilled Nursing Facility Reimbursement and Upcoding," *Health Economics*, accessed February 2017, http://citeseerx.ist.psu.ed u/ viewdoc/download?doi=10.1.1.403.6500&rep=rep1&type=pdf.

The issue with productivity and therapy minutes may be exclusive to therapists, but nurses are under similar pressures. I have experienced nurses being pressured to write notes justifying service and making referrals for residents who at other times would never be considered for programming. I have seen residents literally dragged to walk, just to say therapy was attempted for gait training, when it is clear the person would either never walk or wouldn't be considered for gait training at any other time. I have heard and seen of these as well as other services being delivered, despite protestations from residents to be left alone. (It is only fair to mention that on the flip side of this situation, I have also seen families on many occasions request services for their loved ones that may not be in the best interest of the resident due to his or her age or physical, medical, or cognitive status. Despite the explanations and education provided to the contrary, the family members are insistent that the services be provided.)

This is all done for the purpose of increasing revenue, not necessarily for providing benefit to residents. The prevailing argument is that everyone is entitled to be tried for therapy, and any resident can be trialed on a program for two weeks. Most directors of rehabilitation departments will tell therapists, "If you don't really think they need it, then don't pick them up, but if you think you can make any improvement, you should at least try." At other times therapists are just handed a list of residents for evaluation who are expected to be picked up for therapy.

Furthermore, as the CMI period approaches, there are times therapy services are delayed so therapy minutes can be captured during that period. I have also experienced being cajoled to keep a resident on a program longer than needed so that the minutes could be captured during that period.

An example of how these scenarios play out may best be described by my own recent experience: I wanted to take V. B. off program because the resident was no longer making progress, and there were no additional goals to pursue. I was told this: "Her book [MDS] is due in another week and a half. Can't you find a way to keep her on until next Tuesday?" Another time I was told the following: "You picked up two people for therapy this week who we already got for CMI, and we only have two weeks left." The implied message was clear: "We need you to pick up residents who we need for Case Mix right now. You can think about anyone else later."

Facilities sometimes use strategies to ensure that any potential resident can be captured for Case Mix, so the facility can achieve the highest possible reimbursement rate. These may include but may not be limited to the following:

* Having weekly Case-Mix meetings. In these meetings residents with approaching MDS due dates are reviewed. Their RUG score is reviewed, and they are discussed to determine whether there is any change in their status or any possible changes in function would warrant evaluation for rehabilitation services. While on the surface this seems as though it would be beneficial for the resident, it is being prescribed in a time frame that is based on it being financially beneficial.

☞ Providing the necessary education so that each IDT member understands the principles of CMI in an effort to encourage reporting any resident who could be screened by OT/PT or speech/language therapy (ST) for potential services.

☞ Facilities may conduct rounds or a similar process in which key members of the IDT go around the facility with MDS due-date lists in hand to review and identify residents for changes in condition that would warrant nursing, medical, or therapy intervention.

☞ Having an internal audit system to ensure accurate coding on the MDS. Caregivers sometimes undercode ADLs because of a limited understanding of the difference between limited and extensive assistance. Residents requiring more assistance would obviously be coded for a higher level of care.

☞ Writing progress notes to document changes that would warrant intervention is an essential duty of nurses. There is usually a process in place to ensure that this occurs and that there is an effective, traceable referral communication system between nursing and rehabilitation. This is to ensure the referral does not appear arbitrary, calculated, or capricious. This allays any concerns in the event of a potential audit. If the facility is audited and documentation is reviewed and determined to be satisfactory, there isn't follow-up with the resident to ensure that the situation is described accurately, and there is no oversight to determine if the therapy was actually warranted.

* Conducting weekly meetings where Medicare Part B and Medicaid residents are discussed.
* Ensuring that the result of specialized meetings regarding resident conditions is communicated in a timely fashion to the nurse assessor or MDS coordinator (e.g., skin concerns/changes/breakdowns, weight loss, falls, restraints, behavior). These are all conditions or situations that would be potential referrals for medical, nursing, or therapy intervention and could potentially be captured for CMI.

Rehabilitation-therapy services are weighted heavily in determining the RUG category into which the resident is placed. However, every MDS has a RUG level that also reflects the health and functional level of the resident (also known as the acuity level). This takes into account medical and nursing treatments and interventions. A crucial component of that score is how the resident performs regarding ADLs.

Brief Synopsis of the Case-Mix Categories

A. Rehabilitation—Levels range from ultrahigh intensity to low intensity, which is determined by the number of therapy minutes the resident receives.
   1. Ultrahigh—720 minutes of therapy
   2. Very High—500 minutes of therapy
   3. High—325 minutes of therapy

4. Medium—150 minutes of therapy

5. Low—45 minutes of therapy

B. Nursing Levels—These are the levels of nursing care that are considered pertinent to the resident's medical condition.

1. Extensive Services—Care for a resident with a tracheostomy for ventilator/respirator care, isolation for infection, IV medications, and parenteral feeding or IV fluids.

2. Special Care—Care for a resident with multiple sclerosis, cerebral palsy, Parkinson's disease, or quadriplegia with certain ADL scores; who has experienced respiratory failure or received oxygen, respiratory therapy, radiation, or dialysis; who has pressure ulcers or wounds, a surgical wound, or open lesion that requires treatment; who is tube feeding with aphasia or has fever with dehydration, vomiting, pneumonia, or weight loss.

3. Clinically Complex—There are many clinical conditions that qualify under this category. The facility can also receive credit for a resident having symptoms of depression. Qualifiers include pneumonia, foot wounds, internal bleeding, dehydration, burns, tube feeding, coma, septicemia/sepsis, transfusions, chemotherapy, hemiplegia, or hemiparesis with certain ADL scores, dialysis, oxygen, insulin-dependent diabetes mellitus (IDDM), and physician visits and orders.

4. Impaired Cognition—Impaired cognition includes situations where the resident has a problem being understood, short-term memory issues, or other

cognitive-skills impairment and is coupled with the individual scoring at certain levels on certain measures.

5. Behavior Only – A specific score with additional qualifiers, that take into account hallucinations or delusions and wandering behavior, physical or verbal behavior directed toward others, inappropriate behavior not directed toward others, or resistance to care.

6. Reduced Physical Function Only—This includes reduced physical function that does not meet any criteria for any of the other categories. Restorative nursing programs impact these categories. A restorative nursing program is a nursing intervention program that is intended to assist the individual in functioning as independently and safely as possible. There are eleven categories that are considered for the restorative nursing program.

    1. Passive range of motion
    2. Active range of motion
    3. Assistance with splints/braces
    4. Dressing/grooming
    5. Eating/swallowing
    6. Bed mobility or walking
    7. Transfers
    8. Communication
    9. Amputation/prosthesis care
    10. Urinary
    11. Bowel/toileting

C. ADL Assistance—This includes eleven categories, seven of which are walking in room, walking in corridor, locomotion (e.g., getting around with the use of a wheelchair) on the unit, locomotion off the unit, dressing, personal hygiene, and bathing. The remaining four categories are considered "late-loss." (This term refers to the fact that these are usually the functions that are lost late in the process of the decline.)

D. Bed Mobility—This refers to how the patient moves in bed or other sleep furniture (turns side to side, moves top to bottom or bottom to top, moves from a lying to a sitting position, uses trapeze or side rails to maneuver, any repositioning in bed). An example of limited assistance may include placing a resident's hand on the side rail or guiding an arm or leg into position while the person is turning. Extensive assistance would be lifting the trunk or upper body while the resident pushes up with the feet, lifting or turning even one leg or arm, and using a turn sheet when repositioning.

E. Transfer—This refers to how the resident moves between surfaces and includes transfers to or from the bed, the wheelchair, another chair, gurney to bed, and includes sitting to standing. Limited assistance in this category may even include merely guarding or steadying the resident while a transfer is being made. It may also include use of a light-gait belt during transfers and lifting while the resident pivots or lifts a leg to position.

F. Eating—This refers to how the resident eats and drinks, regardless of skill level. It includes tube feeding, total parenteral nutrition, and IV fluids for nutrition or hydration. A limited assist during eating could be considered placing a cup in the resident's hand or guiding the hand to use a utensil or pick up food. If one has to lift or guide the resident's hand and arm to the mouth to facilitate eating or feed any part of the meal, it would be considered extensive assist.

G. Toilet Use—This refers to how the resident uses the toilet room, commode, bedpan, or urinal and includes transfers on and off the toilet, cleaning self after elimination, managing colostomy or catheter, and managing clothing. If the resident needs help pulling up underwear or pants, it is considered limited assistance. If he or she requires even minimal assistance getting off the toilet or bedpan, it would fall in the limited-assistance category. Supporting any of the resident's weight while the person gets off the toilet or bedpan, requiring the staff to get pants on or off, or inability to assist with any cleaning tasks following elimination would result in extensive assistance being coded.

The performance measures that determine the ADLs examine what the resident actually did each time he or she performed the activity; it does not record what the person might be capable of doing. Coding the degree of support the staff provided during each activity is also relevant. There are six levels of self-performance and five levels of support that are considered when scoring the ADLs.

Self-Performance Codes—How the Person Performs on the Unit

1. Independent—No help or oversight from staff
2. Supervision—Oversight, encouragement, or verbal cuing
3. Limited assistance—Assistance in the form of guided maneuvering of limbs or non-weight bearing assistance
4. Extensive assistance—Weight-bearing assistance
5. Dependent—Full-staff performance
6. Activity does not occur

ADL Support Codes—Degree of Assistance from Others

1. No setup or physical help from staff
2. Setup only
3. One-person physical assist
4. Two-person (or more) physical assist
5. Activity did not occur

From this partial overview of the process for Medicaid reimbursement during CMI for residents in a long-term stay at a skilled-nursing facility, one can clearly see it is complex—possibly even more complicated than that for a hospital stay. There are specific formulas and time frames regarding the number of days and frequency that these services and treatments must be provided in order to qualify for each category. A salient point to remember is that all information related to any of these areas must be documented in nursing notes, addressed in care plans, and correctly coded on the MDS to form a cohesive and accurate picture of the resident. It may be worth considering requesting a copy of each of these documents in order to determine if the resident's status is being accurately presented in this process.

One can view the *RAI Manual for MDS 3.0*, Chapter 6, for a detailed description of each of these categories, the formulas, and specifications at:

https://www cms.gov/Medicare/Quality-Initiatives.../MDS-30-RAI-Manual-V113.pdf.

This website offers replacement pages that have been updated as of August 2017 and will become effective October 2017: www.aanac.org/Information/RAI-Manual.

As of this writing, it is clear there is much work to be done to improve the transparency, reduce the complexity, and somehow remove the profit motive from the process.

● ● ●

Patient Privacy Violation versus Administration Demands and CMI Gain

I worked in a 240-bed facility with an active unit for ventilator-dependent patients as well as a step-down unit for trach patients once they were off the ventilator. When I began working in the facility, there were two part-time speech therapists who shared the position, carrying a minimum number of patients. I began working full time and customarily developed a robust program that varied between fifteen and eighteen patients or residents. By the end of the first year, both administration and ownership acknowledged my outstanding work by giving me, for the first time in my career, a gift for the holidays.

Subsequently there was a dramatic decrease in admissions. At one point the facility had a staggering thirty empty beds. With CMI drawing near, I approached administration to address the fact that the increased number of empty beds was certainly impacting the speech program. The administrator assured me the facility was well aware of the situation.

Fast forward to a few days before the end of CMI. I received a surprising phone call from the administrator—particularly surprising because she was a Jewish Orthodox woman who was calling me on a Saturday. She said the owner wanted me to pick up 5 people for CMI who could use alternative communication and towards then end she had five iPads delivered to the facility. She said I was to go to the facility, find five people who would be candidates for the iPad, and put them on program to capture them for CMI.

I told her I had considered iPad usage in the facility in the past but had encountered two problems. One was that the facility had not been willing to purchase the iPads; the second issue was that there were issues with Wi-Fi in the facility. It had taken so long for administration to supply the iPads and address the Wi-Fi issue that the two patients I had thought were candidates had been discharged.

Her response was that the owner really wanted me to find patients and use the iPads. I agreed to go to the facility on Sunday to look into the matter but reiterated the Wi-Fi issue. Her response was unbelievable—she told me that since there was active Wi-Fi in the lobby, I could treat the patients there. I was horrified. Treat patients in a lobby of a facility—what about HIPAA compliance? Are there no limits to the lengths to which ownership and administration would go to ensure a higher CMI score?

I could not find any suitable candidates for use of the iPad but did identify two additional residents who experienced a change of status and might be able to benefit from a trial of speech therapy.

When the administrator and I met on Monday, I explained my findings: my best clinical judgment was that there were no suitable candidates for using the iPad, but there were a couple of other residents who seemed to have a change of status that would warrant evaluation and treatment. She told me the owner was only interested in the patients who could use the iPads that she purchased.

I was so appalled that I left the facility early. A couple of hours later, I received a phone call from the director of rehabilitation saying that administration wanted to speak with me, and I should drive back to the facility. I lived a distance away in another state, and I had already gone in on a Sunday in an effort to meet their expectations. I decided I would not drive back that day.

From that time on, I became a persona non-grata at the facility. After the appreciation and accolades for a job well done I had received for an entire year, I was both saddened and disappointed—personally and professionally. I began looking for another position and left shortly thereafter.

Delaying Discharge for Case Mix

I was present when the social worker reported to the director of the rehabilitation department that R. D. was scheduled to be discharged home on July 18. The director asked if the patient's discharge could be held until July 26 so the facility could get the patient for Case Mix, because he had already lost a few residents and didn't want to lose another one. The social worker replied that the patient really wanted to go home, and there was no other reason to keep her in the facility. She said, "She's just sitting here doing nothing." The rehabilitation department director was visibly disappointed; the social worker assured him there were two other patients they could keep in the facility who could be captured for CMI.

While the social worker successfully advocated for this patient's discharge, there are many other cases where either the social worker or director of rehabilitation gives the patient some convoluted explanation, essentially a distorted version of the truth, as to why discharge has to be delayed. The patient who is unaware of his or her rights or does not understand his or her condition oftentimes has no choice but to believe the explanation.

Illness versus CMI

My patient became extremely ill and was no longer capable of participating in therapy. I informed the rehabilitation department director that I was going to discharge the patient from program. He asked me if I could postpone the discharge but I explained that her condition had changed significantly and that I was not sure if she would even make it through to the end of the week. He asked me if I thought she would survive through the weekend so she could be captured on her Assessment Reference Date for CMI.

The State Survey Process and Nursing-Home Star Ratings: A Flawed System

● ● ●

Department of Health Annual Survey—A Schedule of Convenience

The head cook in a kitchen told me about a department of health survey visit that started the Monday of Christmas week. I had already been told by the food-service manager that the survey team did not want to be in the facility right before Christmas. The cook went on to tell me the environmental inspector walked through the kitchen with her head toward the ceiling, not looking the slightest bit at the surroundings—although she did notice a lightbulb that was out in an office area. It was his impression that she did not want to find anything that would warrant the team having to spend time with a write-up or find an infraction that might require them to stay longer. The original intended survey was five days; the team left after four days so as not to be in the facility on the Friday before Christmas; the facility was found to be free of deficiencies.

Star Rating

I worked in the facility for a very short time; I left because of the deplorable conditions but I had colleagues who continued working there. Within a few years, I learned that hefty fines had finally been levied against the owner of that facility for a variety of deficiencies, among them were serious safety and cleanliness situations as well as poor resident care. However, the facility had a high star rating.

From Satisfied to Dissatisfied

A staff member recounted her conversation with C. M., a woman who had been a patient in a large, well-known skilled-nursing facility. She said that when she had been a patient there six years earlier, she felt well taken care of, safe, and secure. The facility was a five-star-rated facility at that time, and it was deserved. However, this time her feelings were totally different. She reported she didn't know what happened; the quality of the care, the food, and the overall atmosphere of the place had drastically changed, and it was now more like a three-star facility.

She felt the staff had become sloppy, less interested, and inattentive, and their response times were too long due to the obvious reduced staffing levels. She was concerned that her health and well-being would be compromised if she stayed. This conversation occurred on a Friday, after having been admitted just three stays earlier. By the following Tuesday, she had been discharged to another facility.

This is what happened—only one month prior to this conversation, the facility had been purchased by a large, corporate entity. What was most interesting to me and a fellow speech pathologist was how the facility had achieved a five-star rating in the first place. The nursing staff seemed less than knowledgeable and attentive in a wide variety of areas, there were situations in which long-term care residents' worsening conditions went unnoticed, lingering conditions went unattended, the doctors seemed disinterested, there were a considerable number of food consistency errors, and we heard more than once that "this happens all over." This did not strike either of us as consistent with a five-star rated facility.

Star Rating and Cleanliness

A nurse colleague was telling me about a large, well-known facility in the area in which she worked. One day she went to the ladies' room and found a cockroach crawling on the wall in full view. She took a picture of it and showed it to me. According to her this was not an isolated occurrence at this facility. Cleanliness was a serious issue, and there were many instances of insects throughout the buiilding. As she pointed out, what was most incredulous was that this facility had a five-star rating.

Cost versus Safety

A colleague recounted a situation in a facility that was purchasing cheaper G-tubes. Enteral feeding tubes, or G-tubes, usually require periodic replacement. Long-term use can result in the tube's deterioration, damage, or dislodging. At this particular facility, because the cheaper version was so easily dislodged, the facility administration opted to use Foley catheters to replace the G-tubes, which are considerably less expensive.

The use of a Foley catheter as a replacement for a G-tube—other than as a temporary, emergency measure—is, according to the product literature, an unlicensed use of the product. Additionally, there are other considerations regarding "consent, ethics, and professional responsibilities."[59] This facility, too, has a five-star rating.

Choosing a Facility from a Distance

While attending a professional seminar I met a gentleman; as the conversation ensued I began talking about the professional environs in which I worked. As soon as I mentioned skilled nursing facilities he told me about his father who lived in Florida and needed rehabilitation after breaking his hip. The family decided to look for a suitable short-term rehabilitation setting. He recounted the pains the family went through conducting a search, finally locating a 5-star facility not far from where his father lived. His son wasn't able to make it down to Florida prior to his father's hospital discharge, but planned a trip within a few days of his father's placement in the skilled nursing/rehabilitation facility.

He recalled that, upon visiting his father at the facility, he was appalled by the conditions. His father was unkempt and the surroundings were deplorable., He described that the staff was scarce, inattentive and rude. As a result, within 3 days of his arrival he found a much more suitable short-term placement and transferred his father out of that "5-star" facility.

● ● ●

---

59 O. Ojo, "Problems with Use of a Foley Catheter in Enteral Tube Feeding," PubFacts, accessed May 2017, https://www.pubfacts.com/detail/24732987/Problems-with-use-of-a-Foley-catheter-in-enteral-tube-feeding.

IN THE JUNE 24, 2016, *USA TODAY* "Money" section, the headline below the fold read "Wall Street Banks Ace Fed's Severe Stress Test." [60]As encouraging as this headline may seem, one need only to open the first page and see the headline at the top of the left-hand page to find the irony: "Bank of America Fined $430M for Cash Misuse."[61]

This disparity caught my attention as it relates to the annual state survey process for skilled nursing facilities and the star-rating system. I have personal experience with and knowledge of facilities that are listed as five-star that function in a way that has led me to ponder how that could be possible. They pass their annual state survey every year, some without even a single mention of an infraction. While the notion of a star-rating system intuitively seems like it would be a measure of conveying quality of care and services to the public consumers of health care, it is not necessarily functioning in the way it was originally intended.

My personal experience is in New York State, but there are certainly reports around the country on blogs, websites and in newspapers of nursing homes that passed their respective state surveys only to have later been found with egregious deficiencies and poor quality of care. There is also a website updated monthly (see appendix) that adds facilities to the federal watch list, naming those with the most egregious deficiencies and that provide the worst care.

---

60 M. Krantz "Wall Street Banks Ace Fed's Severe Stress Test" *USA Today Money Section B* June 24, 2016 p.1

61 K. McKoy "Bank of America fined $430M for Cash Misuse" *USA Today Money Section B* June 24, 2016 p.2

These types of discrepancies moved Illinois—on January 1, 2016—to become the sixth state to pass a law allowing cameras to be placed in patients' rooms as a means of chronicling care and ensuring there is no mistreatment or abuse.[62]

While the nursing-home industry is heavily regulated by both federal and state regulatory bodies, the GAO acknowledges that the annual inspections by the department of health in each state "tend to understate the number of serious nursing home problems that present danger to residents."[63] The article continues to state that a report issued in September 2008 indicated that 90 percent of nursing homes received citations for deficiencies that fell in the categories of health or safety in 2007 and that in 17 percent of the facilities those deficiencies fell in the category of "actual harm or immediate jeopardy to patients."[64] In actuality between 1997 and 2010 there were more than twenty reports issued by the GAO that cited substandard care in many nursing homes, understated (serious) deficiencies by state surveyors during annual surveys, unenforced sanctions for resident harm, and both ineffective and inconsistent oversight by the federal government, all of which obviously were

---

62 E. Mongan, "Illinois Becomes the Fifth State to Allow Cameras in Nursing Home Rooms," *McKnights: The News You Need*, accessed August 2015, http://www.mcknights. com/news/illinois-becomes-fifth-state-to-allow-cameras-in-nursing-home-rooms/artic le/434524/?webSyncID=2a2109e8-d644-2377-448a-0398bb1508d7&sessionGUID=2c8 a31c4-ad18-09e7-58c5-12b202da724d.

63 "Nursing Home Residents at Risk," The Long-Term Care Community Coalition, accessed June 2017, http://www.ltccc.org.

64 R. Pear, "Violations Reported at 94% of Nursing Homes," *New York Times*, September 29, 2008 accessed February 2017, www.nytimes.com/2008/09/30/us/30nursing.html

not protecting the health, safety, and welfare of nursing-home residents.[65]

An example of flaws in the system was reported on the ProPublica website as it relates to an egregious situation related to poor care at a particular New York facility. Despite the record of "repeat fines, violations, and complaints for deficient care in recent years,"[66] the founders of the organization that had that facility under its umbrella had been allowed to continue buying nursing homes, placing the organization at the top of the list of that state's largest networks of nursing-home ownership. Prior to buying additional facilities, proposed buyers are to undergo a state-character-and-competence review to ensure that the other health-care facilities owned by the prospective buyer have a record of high-quality care.[67]

How can this happen when there are state oversight agencies conducting annual reviews and charged with identifying and reporting those issues? The agency charged with the final decision in these deals is the Public Health and Health Planning Council, which consists of appointed individuals—many of whom have direct ties to the health-care industry.

---

65 W. Ochinko, "Nursing Home Quality: Findings from GAO Reports," National Health Policy Forum, accessed August 2017, http://www.nhpf.org/library/handouts/Ochinko.slides_03-25-10.pdf.

66 A. Abramo and J. Lehman, "How N.Y.'s Biggest For-Profit Nursing Home Group Flourishes Despite a Record of Patient Harm," ProPublica, last modified October 27, 2015, accessed October 2016, https://www.propublica.org/article/new-york-for-profit-nursing-home-group-flourishes-despite-patient-harm, (hereafter cited as "How N.Y.'s Biggest For-Profit Nursing Home Group Flourishes Despite a Record of Patient Harm").

67 R. Mullman, "Sentosa Care's Expansion in NY," Abuse and Neglect, Advocacy, Staffing and Trial Themes, accessed October 2016, http://www.gpoliakoff.com/.

It is within the council's jurisdiction and authority to urge prospective nursing-home buyers to improve quality of care within their existing homes, but an examination by ProPublica into many of these transactions in recent years shows that this is not happening. Furthermore, the council is supposed to have the Department of Health's character-and-competence recommendation prior to making the decision. A departmental report of one of the principal owners of that company and his partners found that the facilities offered a "substantially consistent high level of care," which is the necessary requirement to receive approval. The company received this commendation despite the fact that records indicate twenty fines have been paid to the federal government in fifteen of the facilities under that company's ownership umbrella just since 2013. There was no mention of the infractions or the payment of these fines in the commendation.

The owners and their relatives and/or associates also applied for ownership in many facilities in 2014. To date they reportedly have ownership shares in over thirty facilities inside and outside of New York State. There are reports that in over a dozen cases the department reported that there were "no repeat violations," yet there were many instances in which this organization's nursing-home facilities were cited on multiple occasions for repeated serious deficiencies.[68]

ProPublica reviewed many nursing-home deals besides those of this particular company and found a green light was given to deals despite a firm statement in the rules that deals shall not

---

68 "How N.Y.'s Biggest For-Profit Nursing Home Group Flourishes Despite a Record of Patient Harm."

be approved when facilities have repeat violations where substandard or poor care places residents at risk. The interpretation that is often applied to give the stamp of approval to these deals is that approval can be granted if the violation or deficiency is not identical or if the facility addressed the deficiency in a timely fashion.

"Advocates for nursing home patients say that instead of a backstop, New York's approval process has become a rubber stamp. The law establishes mechanisms for at least a moderate review of an applicant's character and competence," said Richard Mollot, director of the LTCCC in New York. "The failure to provide complete information on a provider's past performance fundamentally undermines the review process.[69]

In a recent report, Mollot states that the Department of Health, which is a regulatory agency charged with nursing-home oversight in New York State, has "one of the nation's lowest rates of citing nursing home operators for deficiencies in care."[70]

THE STATE SURVEY PROCESS

The CMS is a federal regulatory body that sets forth the parameters for the survey process. The process is carried out by the department of health, which is the overseeing body for nursing-home facilities in each state, and its findings are subsequently reported to CMS. In order for skilled nursing facilities

---

69 "How N.Y.'s Biggest For-Profit Nursing Home Group Flourishes Despite a Record of Patient Harm."

70 R. Mollot, "Executive Summary: Safeguarding Residents and Program Integrity in NY State Nursing Homes," The Long-Term Care Community Coalition, last modified 2015, accessed September 2017, http://nursinghome411.org/?s=safeguarding.

and nursing facilities to receive Medicare and Medicaid reimbursement, they must be found to be in compliance with CMS guidelines. In New York State, the Department of Health oversees nursing homes through its Division of Nursing Homes and Intermediate Care Facilities for Individuals with Intellectual Disabilities Surveillance. This division is the agent that acts on behalf of the federal government's CMS, which monitors quality of care in nursing-home facilities.

Surveys are conducted annually, within a period of up to fifteen months from the previous survey. They are unannounced, and surveyors may arrive at a building at any time. However, it should be noted that most facilities carefully follow the whereabouts of survey teams in their area, so the facility can gauge when the team may arrive. The predictability of the approximate timeframe of when the survey team will arrive has been mentioned in the literature as a source of concern. Though I have seen survey teams arrive in the very early morning hours (six to seven o'clock) and sometimes on a Friday, they more typically arrive on a Monday or Tuesday and conclude their visit by the end of that week.

Once the survey team arrives, the survey team leader is announced to the administrator of the building, who in turn notifies each department head that the department of health state survey has begun. That buzz extends throughout the building like wildfire, and each staff member is on high alert. Once the survey begins, there are signs posted announcing the beginning of the survey process and the dates and duration of the visit. At any point during the state's visit, any concerned person within the building—whether it be staff, a resident, or a family member—is free to speak with the surveyors of the team about any concern. It should be noted, however, that this is rarely done out of fear of repercussions or reprisals.

In the areas with which I am familiar, for the most part the survey teams have remained fairly constant thereby creating a propensity to develop friendly relationships with key administrative staff members within the building. Furthermore, some of these same survey-team members are regular investigators that may be called to a building throughout the year to investigate complaints. Thus, they may overlook or possibly avoid some areas of concern or tip off administration about potential concerns, so corrective measures can be taken to avoid being cited. Some of these infractions may be extremely minor or based on inconsequential technicalities (e.g., a missing signature on a document or the number of inches a box is from a ceiling in a storage area), while others may be more serious.

Many facilities conduct a mock survey in preparation for the actual survey process. I know of an owner of three facilities who hired a former state surveyor as a full-time consultant for one of his buildings after the surveyor left the department of health. The purpose was not only for survey preparation and readiness—uncovering areas of concern and developing and implementing a strategy for correction—but also because of the relationship this past surveyor had with current survey team members. Unsurprisingly this facility passes surveys with few or no infractions or deficiencies.

The survey has been a twofold process: A Life Safety Code (LSC) survey, which is more environmental in nature, and a

Standard Survey. The Standard Survey may have consisted of a traditional survey and a quality indicator survey (QIS). CMS was in the process of transitioning from the traditional survey process, in general terms a more paper based system, to a Quality Indicator Survey (QIS), which was based primarily on electronic computerized records utilizing QIS software to synthesize and organize the findings. During this transition both the QIS and the traditional survey were considered to be valid processes to determine facility compliance and the country has been split on which survey process was being used.

In September 2016, in a surprise move, CMS announced a new nursing home survey process which is touted as being more person-centered. The new process is scheduled to be introduced in three phrases over a 3-year period. Phase 1 (November 2016) included very minor changes to the existing requirements; Phase 2 slated to become effective November 28, 2017 (to include all Phase 1requirements); and finally, Phase 3 which will include the above 2 phases and become effective November 28, 2019. The new survey was designed to incorporate the best elements from the Traditional (original) Survey and the newer QI survey (QIS) process. The latter, because of reliance on computer-based information, was determined to be rigid and inflexible.

In an effort to understand how the new process differs from the QI survey, as well as to understand those aspects of QIS that the new survey process incorporates and a framework of the entire survey process, this chapter will cover much of the information from the QIS process.

The QI survey is conducted in two stages. Stage one consists of analyzing data offsite, based on electronic records transmitted to the state. It may also include information collected by surveyors during on-site observations of the facility, as well as interviews. Once surveyors note particular issues to be of consequence for a particular facility (also known as triggers), the second stage of the process begins. The second stage consists of a systematic investigation of those issues, as well as other areas that are deemed critical for that particular nursing facility. Surveyors may also investigate areas of concern that may not necessarily have triggered but would be considered part of the routine survey process.

Within a short time after the survey team arrives at the facility, it will have asked for and received the following information:

1. A list of important facility personnel and their locations. For example, the team would receive information regarding the administrator, directors of nursing, social services, finance, activities, rehabilitation (and appropriate therapy) staff, the dietitian and food services director or supervisor, charge nurses, pharmacy consultant, medical director, plant engineer, housekeeping supervisor, designated responsible parties for infection control and quality assurance, health-information-management professional, MDS department director and/or personnel, and compliance officer.

2. A copy of the statement of residents' rights that is given to residents.

3. A schedule of meal times, dining locations, and apropos seating arrangements, if necessary, as well as copies of all menus—including therapeutic-diet menus—and a listing of specialized food and/or liquid consistencies that residents receive.

4. Times for medication passes.

5. A list of all admissions during the past month, as well of a list of those residents transferred or discharged within the last three months, including the place of discharge.

6. A copy of the contract between residents and the facility on admission as it relates to Medicare, Medicaid, HMOs, and any other pertinent sources of payment.

7. The layout of the facility in regard to location of nursing stations.

8. The policies and procedures of the facility as they relate to abuse and investigating abuse complaints, as well as the name of the administrator-appointed individual charged with responding to questions to prevent abuse.

9. The facility's policies or procedures to address or monitor accidents, falls, or other incidents and a system to prevent or minimize occurrence of these things. The facility may choose to, but is not mandated to, provide a record of accident or incident reports.

10. Policies and procedures to address noncompliance.

11. Information regarding any resident falling in the fifty-five-or-older-age range.

12. The names of residents who communicate with non-oral communication devices, sign language, other augmentative

communication devices, or hearing aids, as well as those who speak a language that is not the dominant language of the facility.

13. Quality measure or quality indicator reports (QMs or QIs, as they are known), which are markers that identify the existence of potential problems or concerns (or lack thereof) within a facility as they relate to patient-care practices. These practices can affect resident outcomes and may ultimately be reasonable grounds for further investigation. These reports examine residents from both a clinical and psychosocial perspective but are generated solely by in-house nursing-home staff.

QIs and QMs were the outgrowth of a study by both clinicians and research staff at the University of Wisconsin–Madison. The staff developed a set of indicators and the potential risk associated with these indicators, based on clinical research and the guidelines for developing care plans from resident assessment protocols (known as RAPs). Several national interdisciplinary reviews of the data consisted of the following clinical disciplines that are key providers of care in nursing homes: nursing; medicine; pharmacy; medical records; social work; dietetics; physical, occupational, and speech therapy; resident advocates; and administrators. These reviews allowed for critical analysis and helped to refine, define, or delete proposed areas.

In July 1991, the panels that reviewed the information came together to finalize the assessment of the QIs, taking into account input from the various disciplines involved in these independent reviews. An outgrowth of this meeting was an advisory panel charged with researching and analyzing the designated QI areas in greater depth. The advisory panel's result was a set of 175 QI areas, organized into twelve domains.

The twelve domains of the QIs are as follows:

1. Accidents
2. Behavioral and emotional patterns
3. Clinical management
4. Cognitive functioning
5. Elimination and continence
6. Infection control
7. Nutrition and eating
8. Physical functioning
9. Psychotropic drug use
10. Quality of life
11. Sensory function and communication
12. Skin care

There are three essential areas that QM or QI reports cover:

1. Resident versus Facility Level—This includes overall characteristics of the facility. It is a report of the demographics of the resident population within the facility (reported by percentages) as it compares to all other facilities in the state. It includes information on gender, age, payment type/source, diagnosis and pertinent applicable

characteristics, assessment type, condition stability, and potential for discharge.

2. Prevalence versus Incidence—This reports on the status of the facility for each of the MDS 3.0-based quality measures and quality indicators, as compared with both state and national averages.

3. Process versus Outcome—These reports regarding resident levels are samplings that are divided into two categories: chronic care and postacute care. This corresponds to how the residents are divided in the facility QM/QI reports described above. Both reports provide resident-specific information using the CMS MDS 3.0 database.

These areas are examined to determine the following:

a. The number of nursing-home residents who have—or could have—a particular condition.

b. The number of residents in the facility who are observed to have the condition or the percentage thereof.

c. The state or national percentage of residents who have that condition.

d. The percentile ranking of the facility as it relates to overall QM/QI indicators when compared to other facilities in the state. A higher percentile ranking is considered to indicate that the potential exists for a concern regarding the quality of care in the facility.

e. In the event the facility falls above the ninetieth percentile in a particular area (known as a sentinel event), it is flagged by an asterisk.

A sentinel event in the health-care setting is defined (according to the Joint Commission) as "any unanticipated event resulting in death or serious physical or psychological injury to a patient or patients" that is not necessarily related to the natural course of the patient's particular illness. In the most severe of cases, these events may include loss of a limb or loss of gross-motor function but may also include other events where the recurrence would place the patient at risk for a "serious adverse outcome" (e.g., weight loss, dehydration, pressure sores).[71] The Joint Commission has a database to track these events and analyze them to identify "undesirable trends," with the purpose of catching problem areas early and enacting a favorable resolution.

The obvious focus of the survey is to ensure the overall well-being of residents and quality of care administered to them. In addition to the QI report, the survey team reviews Online Survey, Certification, and Reporting data (known by the acronym OSCAR). This data is maintained by CMS in cooperation with the state's long-term-care agencies responsible for surveying nursing-home facilities. Most importantly OSCAR data contains information regarding the history of the facility as it pertains to compliance issues over the past four surveys. This

---

71 "Facts about the Sentinel Event Policy," Joint Commission, last modified February 13, 2017, https://en.wikipedia.org/wiki/Sentinel_event.

information is used to determine if there are patterns of deficiencies in particular tagged areas. The report also lists dates of any complaints that were investigated and federal monitoring surveys over the previous four years. Additionally, the survey team conducts a resident review that is intended to determine the following:

1. How the quality of care and the provision of that care impact resident outcomes and the residents' quality of life in that facility.
2. If the care provided allowed residents to reach or maintain their highest practical physical, mental, and psychosocial well-being.
3. If the facility helps residents achieve the highest-possible quality of life which is determined by sampling a number of residents within the facility. The overall environment, interactions with staff, and services provided to the resident are examined, along with the impact these aspects have on the resident's daily life.
4. If the facility has properly assessed its residents via completing the RAI, including accurate coding and transmission of the MDS to the department of health. Has it also properly assessed resident care needs, conducted and implemented proper care planning, and evaluated the care administered?

In addition to these measures, the survey team conducts interviews both with individuals and groups of residents, attends resident-council and food-committee meetings, interviews pertinent resident or patient family members and friends and legal representatives, as well as the facility ombudsman. These interviews are conducted with the utmost privacy. However, the administration and staff are usually aware of the residents who will be interviewed. Except in rare cases, despite feelings or issues to the contrary, most residents and family members are reluctant to convey adverse events within the facility for fear of repercussions or reprisals, perhaps thinking, "Don't bite the hand that feeds you."

There is a process through which complaints become part of the standard QIS survey process. The survey team leader determines the complaint area and adds it to the list of resident, staff, or facility issues that become part of the standard survey process. The issue is investigated until a decision can be made as to its legitimacy, and the findings are then conveyed to the CMS.

In the event a survey team suspects or identifies substandard quality of care (SQC), it is incumbent upon them to expand the standard survey to more fully investigate the extent of the suspected infractions. SQC is defined as "one or more deficiencies related to resident behavior and facility practices, quality of life, and quality of care, which constitutes immediate jeopardy to resident health and safety."[72] Substandard quality of care can also be defined as widespread deficiencies in either quality of life or quality of care.

If substandard quality of care is found, the administrator is notified and the survey process is extended. This extended

---

72 "Health Facilities Consumer Information Systems Long-Term Care Facility FAQs," California Department of Public Health, accessed May 2017, https://cdph.ca.gov/.

survey is a means to gather any necessary additional information as it relates to nursing and/or medical services and administration in order to determine whether the issues are pervasive or systemic and if they are found to result in a substandard quality of care. Offering substandard care essentially means the facility is noncompliant with the requirements for long-term care as set forth by the CMS.

Federal deficiencies in skilled nursing facilities are rated in terms of scope and severity by how widespread and how flagrant the infractions are. An A-level deficiency is considered to be the minimal level, and L-level is the most severe. A minimal deficiency that may be identified where there is no potential or actual harm for residents may be an omission on a care plan, a document without a signature, or a missing therapy note. The survey team would share these findings, determine the reason for the deficiency, and allow the facility to make the appropriate corrections to avoid such mishaps in the future.

The listing of deficiencies by level and severity are as follows:

* Level 1 (A–C)—This level of deficiency causes no actual harm but may have potential for causing no more than minimal harm or no more than a minor negative impact to the resident.
* Level 2 (D–F)—This is a deficiency that ranges from no actual harm but may result in some level of harm that does not exceed minimal levels as it pertains to the physical, mental, and or psychosocial well-being of the resident. It could also fall into the category of potential harm

that could impact a resident's ability to achieve his or her highest level of well-being across the above-stated areas.

* Level 3 (G–I)—This is actual harm that impacts a resident's ability to maintain and/or reach the highest practical physical, mental, and psychosocial well-being but is not considered to be an immediately jeopardizing situation to an individual resident or the residents at large.
* Level 4 (J–L)—This level places the facility in what is known as Immediate Jeopardy (IJ). The definition of IJ connotes the most egregious violation whereby the facility is not in compliance with long-term-care standards set forth by CMS and that places residents at serious risk for harm, injury, impairment, or death. It assumes the facility has allowed or caused, or is likely to allow or cause, a situation where serious injury, harm, impairment, or death to a resident could occur and/or created or allowed the situation to continue by failing to act to implement preventative or corrective measures. The jeopardizing situation can be a threat to either the physical or mental well-being of the resident and does not necessarily have to be widespread. The finding of IJ is the most severe designation and has serious consequences for a facility.

The consequences of IJ for a facility are as follows:

1. The survey team will remain in the building until it feels the issue has been remedied sufficiently so that it is safe to leave.

2. In the event the situation that created the IJ citation is not corrected while the surveyors are on-site, the facility will immediately be placed on a track to have its Medicare/Medicaid provider agreement terminated within twenty-three calendar days from the last day of the survey. A revised policy for IJ situations proposes that it is up to the discretion of the state's regional survey office (RO) to conduct a revisit to the facility prior to the twenty-three-day deadline to investigate the remediation of the IJ situation rather than conducting a full resurvey process at the end of the twenty-three days.[73] The state may also appoint a temporary manager to oversee the facility with the express purpose of remedying and removing the immediate jeopardy situation.

3. The facility can no longer accept new admissions.

4. A fine is imposed.

The table that follows displays the classes of the various state citations, as well as the criteria needed to classify the level of the citation.[74]

---

73 "Update of State Operations Manual (SOM) Chapter 5, Complaint Investigation," Centers for Medicare & Medicaid Services, last modified April 19, 2013, accessed March 2017, https://www.cms.gov/Medicare/Provider-Enrollment-and-Certification/SurveyCertificationGenInfo/Downloads/Survey-and-Cert-Letter-13-27.pdf.

74 "Long-Term Care Facilities FAQs," Health Facilities Consumer Information System, accessed January 2017, http://hfcis.cdNph.ca.gov/faq/longtermcare.aspx, (hereafter cited as "Long-Term Care Facilities FAQs").

Class	Facility Type	Definition
AA	LTC	<ul><li>Meets the definition of a Class "A" violation</li><li>Was a direct proximate cause of patient death</li></ul>
A	LTC	<ul><li>Imminent danger of death or serious harm to patients</li><li>A substantial probability of death or serious physical harm to patients</li></ul>
B	LTC	<ul><li>Has a direct or immediate relationship to patient health, safety, or security</li><li>Can include emotional and financial elements</li></ul>
Patient Rights B	LTC	<ul><li>Any violation of patient's rights as described in Title 22 of the California Code of Regulations</li><li>A patient's rights violation produces a situation likely to cause significant humiliation, indignity, anxiety, or other emotional trauma but is not serious enough to be a</li></ul>

		Class A, unless CDPH determines such a violation meets the criteria of a Class A.
Abuse Reporting B	LTC	• Failure of the facility to report incidents of alleged or suspected abuse of a facility resident • Must be reported to CDPH immediately or within 24 hours of the incident • Failure of the facility to meet the requirements in Health and Safety Code 1418.91 results in a Class B citation.
Financial Occurrence Reporting B	SNF	• Failure of the licensee to notify CDPH of financial occurrences as described in Health and Safety Code 1421.1 • CDPH must be notified within 24 hours of occurrence. • Notification to CDPH may be in written form if it is provided by fax or overnight mail, or it may

		be communicated by telephone with a written confirmation within five calendar days.
Posting Notice of Imposed Remedies B	LTC	• Facility failure to post notice of remedies imposed for violation(s) of state or federal requirements as described in Health and Safety Code 417.15 will result in a Class B citation.
Written Notice of Imposed Remedies B	SNF	• Written notification of imposed remedies must be given to the following: each resident, each resident's responsible party and legal representative, and all applicants for admission to the facility. • Facility failure to provide written notice of imposed remedies as described in Health and Safety Code 1429.1 will result in a Class B citation.
Posting of Ombudsman	SNF	CDPH shall assess a civil penalty of $100 for each day the facility

Information A & B		fails to post the ombudsman information poster (pursuant to Section 9718 of the Welfare and Institutions Code). • Issued and enforced in the same manner as a Class B citation when the penalty is assessed at less than $2,000 • Issued and enforced in the same manner as a Class A citation when the assessed penalty is equal to or in excess of $2,000
Willful Material Falsification (WMF)	LTC	Any entry in the health-care record that falsely reflects the condition/care/services provided to the resident, such as: • Administration of medication or treatments ordered • Services pertaining to the prevention or treatment of pressure sores or contractures • Tests and measurements of vital signs

		• Notations of fluid input and output
Retaliation/ Discrimination	LTC	Prohibits licensee from discriminating or retaliating against: • Patient • Employee • Any other person who has presented a grievance/complaint or has initiated/cooperated in any investigation/proceeding of any governmental entity relating to care/services/conditions.
C (written as state deficiencies)	LTC	The violation at the time of the occurrence has minimal (remote) relationship to patient health, safety, or security.
Willful Material Omission (WMO)	LTC	• Willful failure to record any untoward event that has affected the health, safety, or security of a patient • Was omitted with the knowledge that the record falsely reflects the

		condition of the patient or care or services provided
Family Council B	SNF	• Facility may not prohibit the formation of a family council • Facility may not limit the function of the family council • Failure of the facility to meet the requirements of Health and Safety Code 1418.4 results in a Class "B" citation.

Deficiencies are classified according to scope and severity on three levels: isolated, pattern, and widespread.

1. Isolated (A, D, G, J)—In an isolated scenario, there is only one resident or a small number of residents affected by one staff member or a small number of staff members. The infraction is limited by location and frequency of occurrence.
2. Scope (B, E, H, K)—Scope is a pattern with an increased number of residents, number of staff, frequency of occurrence, and number of occurrences in multiple locations throughout the facility. It could also refer to one resident being repeatedly affected by the same practice. Though

a pattern emerges, it may not be a pervasive one through-out the facility.

3. Widespread (C, F, I, L)—At this level the deficiencies are pervasive and can potentially cause harm to *all* the residents in the facility or a large percentage of the residents. This level of deficiency is essentially a system failure for a QM area that affects a large number of residents. Repeated issues with lack of heat or air conditioning and inadequate or substandard quality of food are a few examples.

The following chart may provide a clearer understanding regarding isolated, pattern, and widespread deficiencies and how they relate to levels of severity.[75]

---

75 "Long-Term Care Facilities FAQs."

		ISOLATED	PATTERN	WIDESPREAD
LEVEL 4	Immediate Jeopardy to Resident Health or Safety	J	K	L
LEVEL 3	Actual Harm that Is Not Immediate Jeopardy	G	H	I
LEVEL 2	No Actual Harm with Potential for More Than Minimal Harm that Is Not Immediate Jeopardy	D	E	F
LEVEL 1	No Actual Harm with Potential for Minimal Harm	A	B	C

With the exception of an IJ, once the survey process is completed, the survey team gathers to compile its report. An exit conference is held, informing administration and key administrative staff of the findings, and a report of the findings is sent to the facility within two weeks of the exit conference. In the event there were deficiencies that require correction—any or all with a higher than A rating—the facility must file a plan of correction with the department of health within sixty days of receiving the list of deficiencies. Often this plan of corrections—which will give a detailed account of the steps and measures the facility took to address the deficiencies—is the only requirement the state imposes.

Potential areas that may be included in the plan of correction include, but are not limited to, the following:

1. The facility's review, revision, or development of policies and/or procedures to address the areas of concerns
2. The provision and use of new equipment, as necessary
3. Providing staff training to assure ongoing compliance for the implementation and use of new and/or revised policies, procedures, and/or equipment, especially with new and/or temporary staff
4. Additional staffing, changes in assignments, or deployment of staff, as needed
5. A method to monitor changes and to ensure that those changes being made are supervised, evaluated, and reinforced by responsible facility staff

Deficiencies that fall into the following categories are supposed to result in a fine being levied against the facility:

1. All IJ and SQC events—deficiencies rated as F, H, I, or J–L in one of the following areas: resident behavior and facility practices, quality of life, or quality of care
2. Two or more G deficiencies in the same survey (Double G)
3. Any G deficiencies where a G or greater deficiency was cited within the prior two survey cycles and continues to be present in the facility

Fines are determined and assessed by the state pursuant to public health law. In New York State, the fine is determined by the Department of Health's Office of Health Management Systems Division of Quality and Surveillance for Nursing Homes, which creates what is known as an enforcement packet that includes recommendations for specific fine amounts. The legal department to which the fines are submitted then negotiates a settlement with the nursing home in question, and the fines are ultimately finalized in what is known as Stipulation and Orders. When considering the amount of the fine, the facility's history of compliance or noncompliance is taken into consideration.

However, a report from the State of New York's Office of the State Comptroller found that the bureau's legal department routinely did not assess any fines for citations falling in the range of minimal harm, regardless of the facility's past performance. The alternative was an accepted plan of correction.[76]

The report goes on to state that for the past seven years, the time between the survey end date—when the deficiencies were first identified and reported—and the date of fines being imposed has been steadily increasing (a period of up to 3.89 years, and there have been some cases stretching up to six years). At the same time, the number of fines and total amount of imposed monetary fines peaked several years ago and has been on a steady decline—amounting in many cases to no more than a slap on the wrist. One can easily conclude that when the distance between the identified problem and the enforcement action increases, the deterrent effect is minimized. The poor practice or noncompliant situation more than likely continues and may grow in both scope and severity.

Prior to 2008, as per Section 12 of the New York State Public Health Law, the maximum amount of fine imposed was a mere $2,000 per incident for the most serious infraction, including those that fell into the IJ category. An amendment to that law was added in 2008 that included additional fines for particular types of violations (i.e., $5,000 for repeat fined violations in consecutive years—in this way repeat violations that were previously unfixed would not incur this additional levied amount) and increased the fine for noncompliance resulting in serious physical

---

76 T. P. DiNapoli, "Nursing Home Surveillance," Office of the New York State Comptroller, accessed October 2016, https://www.osc.state.ny.us/audits/allaudits/093016/15s26.pdf, (hereafter cited as "Nursing Home Surveillance").

harm to $10,000. This is still a negligible amount, considering the seriousness of the impact on the resident.

Yet these 2008 amended fine amounts were due to expire in April 2017, when there would have been a return to the previous fine amounts: $2,000 regardless of the severity of harm or potential harm to the resident. Though the additional fine amounts have been extended to April 1, 2020, these reduced fines clearly devalue both the importance of the infraction and the importance of the resident. The report calculated that the $2,000 is "less than the equivalent of one week's revenue derived from one bed," as calculated from the estimated average daily rate for a nursing home (ranging from $288 to $407 per bed, per day, depending on the region).[77] How is this an incentive to provide better-quality care?

Furthermore, under the new survey process, in the event a facility is found out of compliance for specific Phase 2 requirements. CMS has indicated they will not enforce civil monetary penalties, denial of payment and/or termination of the Medicare/Medicaid beneficiary agreement for a period of one-year beginning November 2017. They will use this year-long period to educate facilities about specific Phase 2 quality standards by requiring a directed plan of correction or additional directed in-service training. Enforcement for other existing standards (including Phase 1 requirements) would follow the standard process. While there may be specific care quality measures that will be examined and looked at differently or more closely, a one year

---

77 "Nursing Home Surveillance."

moratorium on penalties seems to be waiver to benefit providers rather than a way to ensure improved quality care for nursing home residents which the new survey was designed to address.

The survey team is also charged with investigating the facility for the existence of a functioning Quality Assessment and Assurance (QA) committee, which is charged with identifying issues related to quality of care, and—in the event there is a lack of quality care—it is to determine the cause or reason of the deficiency in a timely fashion and provide and implement corrective measures. The QA committee is supposed to meet, at the very least, on a quarterly basis and consists of the director of nursing services, the medical director or physician designee appointed by the facility, and at least three other staff members that would usually include key-department-head staff (e.g., the director of rehabilitation, dietary, social services, or activities).

Additionally, the committee must evaluate any corrective measures to ensure they are applied and maintained and, if warranted, revise them to ensure consistent compliance, thereby eliminating the possibility of placing other residents at risk as a result of the issues identified. It is important to note that the survey team is not privy to any written material regarding the QA committee but relies on verbal reports that the facility provides to surveyors. I am aware of several facilities that not only do not hold regular QA meetings but do not even have a QA committee. Upon survey key members of the facility agree among themselves what information will be supplied to the survey team. In this way, they can include or withhold information as they see fit.

The final department of health survey report should always be readily available and on view in the hallway of every facility. In addition, the phone number for anonymous reporting of concerns or infractions should be listed throughout the facility. Though it is rarely put into practice, the policy is, "If you see something, say something." Under the new survey process, everyone in the facility is a mandated reporter. Anyone who is witness to, or has knowledge of, abuse of any kind within the facility is obliged to inform local law enforcement.

It appears that the state survey process as an oversight for nursing homes is sufficiently encompassing to identify potential sources of inadequate or poor quality of care that would negatively impact residents and would serve as an acceptable benchmark. Since facilities are audited by state surveying bodies annually—technically every fifteen months—one would not expect to see a facility with extensive egregious failures in its care of residents. It should be rare to see deficiencies escalate to the immediate jeopardy level or to see care so substandard that facilities are placed on a federal watch list.

So why is it that these things are not as uncommon as we would expect? An ABC News article entitled "Report Finds That Lack of Enforcement Allowed for Neglect at State Nursing Homes" that was published on July 26, 2016, may provide some insight.

Pennsylvania Auditor General Eugene DePasquale issued a report that essentially said the Department of Health was remiss in its documentation, adherence to standard protocols, and enforcement, which resulted in neglect and unsanitary conditions in nursing homes to "slip through the cracks."

"What this tells me is the Department of Health was not looking," DePasquale said during a press conference. "And when you don't look, there's no way to discover problems." In the same article, he goes on to say that nursing homes that "failed to meet state standards were often not cited during Department of Health Inspections."[78]

The question is a moral one: why are the regulatory agencies charged with overseeing nursing homes that are supposed to care for our precious elder citizens—our aging parents—not looking? Will a new survey process be the solution to impact the much-needed change in the care of our elder citizens residing in nursing homes and skilled nursing facilities?

THE STAR-RATING SYSTEM

The Nursing Home Compare (NHC) website—see appendix for website address—is a database that lists and ranks all licensed nursing-home facilities throughout the country by ascribing a star-rating system (five stars being the best) in an effort to help consumers determine which facilities to choose for themselves and their loved ones. Facilities on the website can be located by name, as well as by city and state. The website also includes information on ownership and whether a facility is for profit, not for profit, or government owned and operated.

---

78 A. St. Hilaire, "Report Finds that Lack of Enforcement Allowed for Neglect at State Nursing Homes," ABC News, Updated September 2016, accessed November 2016, http://abc27.com/2016/07/26/report-finds-that-lack-of-enforcement-allowed-for-neglect-at-state-nursing-homes/.

Star ratings are ascribed to facilities based on determinations in each of the following three categories:

1. Health-inspections rating—This rating is based on the latest three years of on-site health-department surveys and is supposed to take into account information from both the standard surveys and any other complaint surveys. The most recent inspection report carries more weight than that from previous years.

2. QM rating—The QM rating takes into account information from anywhere between eleven to sixteen physical and clinical measures and does not include information about the facility's use of antipsychotic (psychotropic) medications for both long-term-care residents and short-term patients. This information is also based on data prepared and submitted by the facility itself.

3. Staffing rating—Staff rating has been historically based on *self-reported* information from the facility and takes into account both registered nurse (RN) hours per resident, per day, and total staffing hours per resident, per day, as determined by licensed practical nurses (LPNs), licensed vocational nurses (LVNs), and CNAs and the levels of care needed by the residents of the facility or on a particular unit (e.g., subacute care, clinically compromised, or dementia unit).

This issue was addressed in the Affordable Care Act (Section 6106) which requires a facility to electronically transmit payroll reports of regular, agency and contract staff to their respective state.

The first mandatory reporting period began July 1, 2016 and must be reported by the end of the 45th following each fiscal quarter. The system allows the quantifiable data to be verified and, combined with census information from that facility, can be used to determine actual staffing levels as well as employee turnover and tenure, all of which impact the quality of care. This information can be published and available to the public. The Centers for Medicare & Medicaid services has created a system for reporting of this information known as the Payroll-Based Journal (PBJ).[79]

More detailed information on the star-rating system can be found at the "Five-Star Quality Rating System Technical Users' Guide," in which there is an in-depth description of the ratings, methodology, and calculations.[80] It can be found at:

https://www.cms.gov/Medicare/Provider-Enrollment-and-Certification/CertificationandComplianc/downloads/users-guide.pdf

The NHC database not only contains star-rating information but also contains a downloadable copy of the statement of deficiencies (SODs) for any facility—including the name of the nursing home, date it received the deficiency, tag number,

---

79 "Staffing Data Submission PBJ" Centers for Medicare & Medicaid Services Last modified 9/28/2017 accessed October 2017, https://www.cms.gov/Medicare/Quality-Initiatives-Patient-Assessment-Instruments/NursingHomeQualityInits/Staffing-Data-Submission-PBJ.html

80 "Technical Users' Guide for Nursing Home Compare Five-Star Quality Rating System" January 2017 accessed March 2017 https://www.cms.gov/Medicare/Provider-Enrollment-and-Certification/CertificationandComplianc/downloads/usersguid,e.pdf

scope and severity of the deficiency, and the current status and/ or corrective action for the deficiency. Additionally, the report contains all penalties, including the number, amount, and payment details for any fine associated with the deficiencies that were imposed on a facility.

A facility's staffing rates and ratios, citations, and quality-measure performance may be compared with both state and national averages. When choosing a skilled-nursing facility, it is always wise to make an on-site visit armed with information and a list of pertinent questions specific to your loved one's condition and needs or about the facility in general.

In many instances, however, there is insufficient time to make an on-site visit. Hospitals may inform patients and/or families of an upcoming discharge without much notice, often placing consumers in the position of having to make a hasty decision under extreme pressure. In many cases the patient or family never considered placement in a facility and, therefore, relies on information from either word of mouth or the NHC website, which may not be reliable.

Even more disheartening are the cases where an older, more compromised, patient without family support or advocacy is unwittingly placed in a facility based on availability or marketing. The patient arrives in the facility not knowing where he or she is or how he or she got there; one can only imagine how that must feel. If the facility is one with substandard care practices, there can be strong physical and emotional implications for the patient.

Important Considerations

There are important caveats when considering the NHC star-rating system as a guide for choosing a nursing home. First, one can easily see that the rating system and the survey results are interdependent. The star-rating system, which is so reliant on survey results, is significantly problematic. There are numerous studies, newspapers articles, personal accounts, and blogs regarding the lack of identification or reporting of substandard nursing care—even to the extreme of serious abuse or neglect. Furthermore, the scope and extent of the deficiency are often underrated or in some cases not reported at all.

Second, as with staffing levels that had been self-reported and based on unsubstantiated or unverified information, one can easily see that facility's will shed the most favorable light on the care and attention that will be given to the resident or patient.

QMs are also self-reported and unsubstantiated. Thus, one can assume the nursing home would be inclined to report this information to its advantage. As of 2015 the CMS began implementing improvements affecting reporting of QMs and has added antipsychotic drugging rates to the QM star rating.

One example, as reported in the 2014 *New York Times* article entitled "Medicare Star Ratings Allow Nursing Homes to Game the System," reinforces the problem with the rating system—more specifically, the five-star rating.[81]

---

81 K. Thomas, "Medicare Star Ratings Allow Nursing Homes to Game the System," *New York Times*, August 24, 2014, (hereafter cited as "Medicare Star Ratings Allow Nursing Homes to Game the System").

The article reports that in 2011 Ken Chandler took his elderly mother to the Rosewood Nursing Home—a small, 110-bed facility—in a suburb of Sacramento, California, which had a five-star rating, essentially giving it a "Medicare seal of approval." Rosewood was a picture of opulence and luxury and gave the impression it was deserving of the five-star rating. Consistent with many for-profit nursing homes in recent years, owners moved to renovate the facility—especially lobbies, rehabilitation units, and departments—to convey a luxury, high-end appeal. Rosewood's lobby resembled a luxury hotel with all the accoutrements—high ceilings, leather chairs, and serene paintings of pastoral landscapes—and Chandler and his wife were impressed by the five-star rating and the hotel-like appearance.

Chandler was unaware that, despite Rosewood's five-star rating, it had been fined $100,000 in 2013 for the death of a woman in 2006 that resulted from an overdose of a powerful blood thinner medication. In addition, according to the California Advocates for Nursing Home Reform, from 2009 to 2013 there had been 102 complaints filed against Rosewood; some say the complaints actually numbered approximately 164. Rosewood had also been the subject of about a dozen lawsuits in recent years from patients and their families claiming substandard care.

Ken Chandler placed his mother in Rosewood in 2011, after she had sustained a fall that resulted in a broken femur. Chandler's mother experienced several serious falls while she was a resident at Rosewood and died a few months later. Subsequently the family filed a lawsuit against the facility. The article reported that the family felt misled by the rating system which played a significant role in their choice of Rosewood for their mother. Mrs. Chandler was quoted as saying, "You don't know where to look to get accurate information. I can go and find a preschool for my child better than I can find a skilled-nursing facility for my loved one."[82]

The *Times* article goes on to say that nursing homes, despite having a history of poor care, continue to receive high ratings—especially in areas such as staff and QMs that are self-reported. "Of more than fifty nursing homes on a federal watch list for quality, nearly two-thirds hold four- or five-star ratings for their staff levels and quality statistics."[83]

The percentage of facilities that achieved a four- or five-star rating was 39 percent in 2009; in 2013 that number had risen to 52 percent. Some believe this is related to the transition to the QIS, whereby there are only a limited number of parameters that the surveyors are allowed to examine, as generated by the facility's computer analysis. The computer-determined parameters are stringent, and the team is not permitted to look beyond them, notwithstanding an egregious noncompliance.

There are agencies that track nursing-home star ratings and work with facilities to help them bolster their ratings. The self-reporting of staffing ratios that helped determine the number of stars rated for that category is based on a form the nursing home completes in preparation for its annual state survey.

---

82 "Medicare Star Ratings Allow Nursing Homes to Game the System."
83 "Medicare Star Ratings Allow Nursing Homes to Game the System."

From personal experience in the almost forty homes in which I have worked, I can attest to the fact that staff is has been added intentionally near the time of the inspection. Workers throughout every facility have been aware of it and complain of "working short" until it's time for state inspection. This practice has allowed the facility to complete the paperwork reflecting higher staffing ratios. These false numbers have been reflected in the survey results and reported on NHC, thereby giving the false impression of adequate staffing ratios during the majority of the year.

The same *New York Times* article reported that this is no more evident than in an excerpt of an e-mail that was included in a lawsuit filed this year against Medford Multicare Center, located on Long Island, by the New York attorney general. David Fielding, the nursing home's administrator, wrote about the state survey that "the inspection period is so crucial" that it is like "our Super Bowl" and stated that following the state inspection, staff levels would drop. Fielding went on to write "the staffing hours will be a little high for this week but will drop the following week."

Though the public relies on the NHC website and the star-rating system to make the best choices possible to meet health-care needs, consumers are being misled. One may conclude that the rating system seems to be based on shielding ownership from the repercussions associated with noncompliance and substandard care rather than the protection of the residents entrusted to their care.

Because the new survey process becomes effective November 28, 2017, CMS is freezing the star rating system for a period of 1 year from that date until November 28, 2018 when it is expected the majority of facilities will have been surveyed under the new system. Until that time, information on facility performance will be offered on the NHC website based on survey reports; facilities with serious quality concerns will be flagged.

CMS will provide additional information regarding this matter on the NHC website in the future. In addition, in response to cries for improved transparency of nursing home ownership, NHC has begun to reflect this information when reporting facility deficiencies and poor-quality care. However, there is a greater need for transparency of deficiencies as it relates to nursing home ownership chains.

Information on the new survey process is contained in the Revision to the State Operations Manual (SOM) Appendix PP for Phase 2 which also includes a revised F-Tag system. Some F-tags have been renumbered, others moved or combined consistent with citations for new regulations. An brief overview of selected features of the new LTC survey process will be covered in Chapter 10: New Trends in Nursing Home Reform.

• • •

Cost versus Quality

While working with a resident during a lunch meal, I wanted to trial a soup item. The server for the unit told me that the facility used to provide two soups for each meal—a regular soup and a fortified soup for those who were in need of extra nutrition. Since the new, corporate ownership took over within the past month and a half, most often only one soup was offered—either the regular or fortified version. She explained the reduced kitchen staff no longer had the time to prepare both versions of soup. This begs the question: What about the residents in need of the fortified soup on the days only the regular soup is available? What about those who don't need a fortified soup but receive it anyway on the days only the fortified soup is available? Furthermore, the server told me the soups were not the same quality. There was more water to increase the volume and cornstarch added to enhance the body. This same facility is one in which the lead dietitian informed me of the instructions since the takeover of the facility by the new corporate ownership mandating that $500,000 be cut from the budget.

Cost versus Nutrition—The Importance of Making Your Feelings and Needs Heard

At the aforementioned facility, one could not help but notice that not only had the size of the chicken leg quarters become appreciably smaller, but they were now cut into two pieces so that the leg was separate from the thigh. In the days that followed, the serving sizes also changed: a serving of chicken was now either one small thigh or two small legs. When questioned the server indicated those were the instructions from the kitchen; we all agreed it was horrible. When requested, she acquiesced—under duress—and provided at least a leg and thigh.

Two days later a patient of mine, T. F., expressed his feelings about the reduced chicken portion. He felt insulted that as a grown man who had been living in the facility for a few years, he now had to accept this meager amount of food.

He actually used the word indecent. He went on to say that the woman who was his tablemate at meals felt similarly but was reluctant to say anything about the situation for fear of reprisals.

I urged T. F. to speak up for himself and his tablemate but he was reluctant. I told him it was his right to receive an appropriate amount of food at each meal. We also agreed the serving probably did not measure up to the required four ounces of protein. I asked if I could speak about the matter to the appropriate parties on his behalf. He agreed as long as I did not mention his name, repeating concerns about reprisals.

The next day I had the opportunity to speak with the kitchen supervisor. I acknowledged understanding the facility was newly acquired by a for-profit, corporate entity, but I maintained that the situation with the portion size was ridiculous. As promised I did not mention names, but reported that on one specific unit residents felt it was insulting and downright indecent. The response was that the chicken was now sent in pieces. I replied that while I understood that previously a whole chicken leg quarter per person would serve two people, kitchen staff was now able to stretch the number of people served with the same amount of food to three (i.e., one paltry thigh as one serving, two legs as a second, and another paltry thigh as the third) as a cost cutting measure. Besides being unacceptable in all probability the paltry sized pieces did not meet the required four ounces of protein which might motivate someone to call and report the matter to the state department of health.

The next meal the server informed me instruction from the kitchen was to give each person a leg and a thigh as a serving of chicken.

Cost of Staff Training versus Trach Patient Care (Example 1)

I was asked to work in a facility that had been not-for-profit but had recently been purchased by a major, for-profit corporation. Because of my expertise with ventilator-dependent and tracheostomy patients, the facility administration decided to accept patients who had tracheostomy tubes in place. On several occasions, I urged the administrator to appropriately train staff in tracheostomy care prior to accepting any of these patients. Unfortunately, my counsel fell on deaf ears.

The first tracheostomy patient was accepted without any procedures in place or appropriately trained staff to care for her. The staff scrambled for appropriate emergency bedside equipment but could not get authorization from the corporate office to order from its vendor. In addition, though the facility had no respiratory therapist on staff to assess the patient, administration decided to borrow one from a sister facility located approximately thirty minutes away.

The respiratory therapist visited the patient and recommended a particular type of tubing that would ease discomfort by providing both moisture and oxygen to the patient's airway. The corporate supply company had no knowledge of that particular kind of tubing, and the facility could not get authorization to purchase it from any other vendor. I made some phone calls to respiratory-therapist colleagues and was able to borrow the tubing from a facility where I had worked previously. The central-supply employee was sent to pick up the tubing on the following day.

It did not end there. Since the company could not get authorization for the particular trach tubes the patient required, and by law a spare trach has to be at bedside in case of emergency, I called a supply company with whom I had a good working relationship and personally paid for the emergency bedside equipment which was delivered overnight. The scramble to obtain the necessary equipment to meet the patient's needs was extremely stressful.

I urged the administrator once again to provide appropriate staff training as apparently their understanding and ability to care for trach patients was not up to par. I provided him with the names of two colleagues who were willing and available to provide the necessary training. I continued to follow up with him but *heard nothing about scheduled training, yet the staff continued to lack the appropriate skills to care for the patient.*

He ultimately informed me that the cost of the training was too high. I couldn't believe my ears. The cost of staff training to care for a seriously compromised patient with special needs, for whom the facility was receiving top reimbursement dollars because of her clinically complex condition, was too high! I calculated that the training may have cost approximately Five-hundred dollars. Ultimately the relatively small cost of training took priority over a person's life.

The situation continued. A second trach patient was accepted under similar circumstances, with lack of appropriate life-saving bedside emergency equipment. Staff skills continued to be lacking, and I continued to tell the administrator that the facility was placing the patients' lives in jeopardy.

Finally, a third trach patient was admitted late one afternoon. When I arrived at the facility the next morning I was immediately summoned to the rehabilitation unit. The patient's tracheostomy tube had dislodged and couldn't be reinserted. The staff was frantic and because they knew this was an area of my expertise, looked to me for assistance. They asked me to attempt reinserting the trach tube but I explained that was not within my scope of practice. I advised the nurse who had left the patient's room reporting that "she seemed to be OK" to return and continually monitor the patient's condition, use other emergency procedures as needed to ensure her breathing, and call 911. Ultimately the paramedics arrived and took the patient to the hospital.

I found the administrator to report what had happened; his response to me was, "I guess you're going to tell me 'I told you so.'" I explained that was not the case, but in my experience with trach patients, I knew that sooner or later a circumstance would arise that would require appropriately trained and competent staff to attend to an emergency situation to keep the person alive. That person's family ultimately moved their loved one to a different facility. During the

15 months that I worked at that facility, the administrator never arranged for the staff training. However, I am happy to say they did not admit additional patients with tracheostomy tubes.

Staff Training—Cost versus Trach Patient Quality Care (Example 2)

I encountered a similar circumstance almost 1 year later when I began working at a facility that went from a not-for-profit entity to for-profit ownership. It was purchased by a corporation that owned approximately 40 skilled nursing facilities/rehabilitation centers and other specialized facilities.

When I began working at the facility, there were two residents with long-standing tracheostomy tubes being cared for by obviously poorly trained staff. There were inadequate supplies at bedside and poor infection control standards which would certainly compromise resident's health and well-being. Shortly after my arrival the facility admitted a third patient with a tracheostomy tube. The poorly trained staff and issue with inadequate emergency supplies continued.

My cries for staff training to enhance staff knowledge thereby ensuring and improving quality care were deflected, delayed and finally denied, yet the facility continued to receive reimbursement at a higher rate for the specialty services that were needed to care for the patient.

Once again, the cost of staff training superseded patient care and was of greater importance than a person's life.

Interestingly enough it was the same facility in which the director of admissions told me the central office did not give a rat's ass. One could deduce that appeared to be the case from the decision that was made about the training.

Cost versus Patient Well-Being

I worked in a facility that had recently been taken over by a large, corporate entity that owned dozens of facilities. Within the first couple of weeks, the plastic disposable cups that were used to serve the patients and residents drinks got noticeably smaller and so thin that a healthy person had difficulty holding them, let alone someone frail or infirm. It struck me that the only consideration was the money saved on the amount of liquid being consumed and on the cheaper version of the cup. No consideration was given to the potential negative consequences on a variety of levels: because the cups were so flimsy, they were difficult to hold, which would ultimately increase the occurrence of spills and create more waste; patients and residents could potentially opt to drink less because of the spillage and also consume less because of the smaller cup; and for those who were having a particularly hard time—who otherwise would be able to hold the cup—staff time would be spent having to hold the cup in order for the person to drink. That situation in itself created a more dependent, degrading situation for a capable individual.

Of even greater concern were the conditions created by reduced liquid intake: increased dehydration, urinary-tract infections (oftentimes with associated mental changes or confusion), cost of prescriptions/antibiotics to address infections, and increased hospitalizations. Was the cost of cups more important than the health and well-being of those entrusted to the facility's care?

Medication and Nursing Staff Hours

An NP colleague told me the facility had a meeting with the corporate doctor, who informed the medical team there would now be a maximum number of medications that could be prescribed. Intuitively to me this seemed like a good idea as I have certainly seen patients with orders in excess of twenty medications. However, it was explained that there were specific conditions that might require multiple medications and that, in addition to the vitamin supplements that a patient may need, in many cases one could not help but exceed the designated number of medications.

We went on to discuss that the "official" philosophy was that nurses would have more time for direct patient care. The NP was informed by the doctor who was in charge of the practice that supplied the medical personnel to the building, that by limiting the number of medications a nurse had to dispense, the facility could reduce the number of needed nursing staff hours. Therefore, the purpose was one of a cost-saving measure all the way around, with little regard for patient care.

CHAPTER 8

Facility Staffing and Responsibilities

• • •

Nursing Staffing

An RN colleague of mine recounted a time when she was the evening supervisor (and only RN) on duty in a facility that had several incidents and three admissions while she was on duty. In order to attend to each situation, she needed to rely on assistance from the LPN staff. When this RN supervisor arrived on one of the units where an admission had already arrived, one of her most competent LPNs informed her that, in an effort to help the RN, she had already completed the assessment of the patient.

Despite the fact that the RN was overwhelmed by the number of the situations in the facility and wanted to rely on the assessment of her competent LPN, she felt compelled to examine the patient herself. She was astonished by what she found!

The patient, who was a dark-skinned black man, had fallen and had severe black-and-blue areas on one side of his body, extending from his hip to his mid-thigh. This was readily apparent to her trained eye but was missed by the LPN. She questioned the LPN and admonished her about not documenting the black-and-blue areas on her assessment. The LPN apologized profusely for her egregious error.

This is only one very small example of why it is critical for every facility to have an RN on duty twenty-four hours a day. Furthermore, for the highest level of patient care, this author contends that having an RN on duty twenty-four hours a day should not be limited to one who functions solely as supervisor in an administrative capacity. In this example, if this facility only had an RN on call during that shift and the LPN had called in her assessment, the RN would unwittingly be agreeing to a careless and inaccurate assessment of the patient.

I have RN colleagues who have indicated that these situations are unsafe and pose tremendous liability to their licenses. In a few cases, I have known RN evening supervisors who have informed the director of nurses or administrators that if these situations persist, they will refuse to "take the key" or start a tour.

These staffing decisions are solely financial in nature. Owners' and administrators' primary concerns are cost and profit; patient care and safety do not seem to be considerations in the equation. As long as there are no specific staffing requirements, these situations will prevail.

Staff Cuts versus Customer Service

A facility with which I am acquainted was taken over by a major corporation. Within a short period of time, the changes in staffing ratios were appalling: for the 3:00 to 11:00 p.m. shift, where there were residents with dementia who required heavy care, only two CNAs (down from four) were scheduled for forty patients, and oftentimes only one LPN was scheduled. Families and patients/residents began to complain. Staff nerves became increasingly frazzled, tensions rose, job-related injuries mounted, and the staff became increasingly demoralized.

The only action taken by administration was to begin a series of staff education sessions on customer service—which was essentially tantamount to blaming the staff for the reduced level of care. Once again no one addressed the staff shortage that created the issues. There was apparently no thought given to the increase in falls, incidents, and bedsores, which would undoubtedly result from the facility being understaffed. The staff began to voice their concerns to administration. They were told, "If you don't like it, you know where the door is; submit your resignation and leave."

MD Billing versus MD Visits

I was speaking with a colleague who is an NP. The practitioner explained that the reports written after seeing a patient were countersigned by the doctor who owned the practice for whom she worked. When the note was countersigned by the doctor a higher reimbursement would be received for a doctor visit as opposed to a visit by an NP.

I personally knew the doctor who signed those notes, and that physician rarely visited the facility, except for an administrative meeting. The impression I gleaned from the conversation was that this was not an unusual occurrence.

Cost versus Patient Safety

An NP colleague recounted a situation in which he was approached about to write a note approving a patient be allowed to go to an outside appointment without being accompanied by a staff member. The NP refused, indicating that the patient was prone to falls and it was an unsafe situation. My colleague continued to receive pressure from the administrator and the director of nurses to write the note approving the situation—all this so the facility would not have to pay a staff member for the necessary few hours required for the patient's outside appointment. In order to deflect the situation, the NP suggested that if the physical therapist wrote a note indicating the patient was safe he would reconsider. The physical therapist would not agree that the patient was safe to go to the outside appointment unattended. Ultimately, and begrudgingly the facility paid for a CNA to accompany the patient to the appointment.

● ● ●

Once an individual is placed in a facility, patients/residents and their loved ones will be become acquainted with administrative, medical, rehabilitation, nursing, and supportive staff members who all are part of the IDT. This is a brief synopsis of those team members, the roles they play, and requirements for their respective positions.

Medical

Medical Director

There is usually a head doctor who oversees the medical services in the facility and who is known as the medical director. All doctors fall under his or her supervision. This doctor may or may not provide direct service to patients or residents within the facility. The medical director usually visits the facility a few hours each week but may or may not have a set schedule.

Facility Physician

Each individual admitted to a facility is assigned a staff physician who oversees all services provided to the individual. Doctor's orders are required for all treatments administered. An individual's private-care physician who is not on staff at the facility cannot visit the patient or resident while he or she is an inpatient, although the facility physician may choose to consult with the individual's primary-care physician on an as-needed basis.

The facility physician oversees and makes decisions regarding medications, appropriate specialized tests, and referrals to outside specialists, and this medical professional maintains the ultimate decision as to whether a patient's condition warrants hospitalization. Many physicians are under pressure from administration to refrain from hospitalizing patients unless absolutely necessary. This is especially crucial in the first thirty days following admission, especially if the number of occupied beds of the facility falls below a certain level (also known as the census). In the latter case, the facility does not have bed hold, which means the facility cannot reserve any beds for patients who are hospitalized.

Physician's Assistant and Nurse Practitioner

Many facilities have developed a model with a primary doctor who oversees an individual's care, but an NP or PA attends an individual's everyday needs. Usually the NP or PA is required to complete a certain number of contacts per day for billing purposes. This person is the primary medical contact for the individual and provides a wide range of health-care services, including prescribing medications, ordering special labs and tests, and diagnosing and treating common minor illnesses and injuries.

Nursing

Director of Nurses

Each facility has a director of nursing services who is responsible for, and oversees, all nursing staff activities and duties and has both a clinical and administrative role. Directors of nurses (DONs) are also responsible for ensuring adequate staffing to meet all the patient or resident needs. They must also be able to provide direct patient care on an as-needed basis.

The basic requirements for the position are completion of at least an associate's degree as a registered nurse, passing the National Council Licensure Examination for Registered Nurses (NCLEX-RN), and experience as an RN in a health-care setting. Typically, an RN is expected to have from five to ten years of experience in at least a supervisory or unit-manager role prior to being considered for this position. Many of those interested in achieving the position of DON pursue a bachelor's degree in nursing. Some facilities require the DON to also hold a master's degree in nursing, while still others opt for someone who also has a degree in nursing and healthcare administration or even business administration.

Some facilities, but certainly not all, hire an assistant director of nurses (ADN or ADON) who provides further assistance to the DON in both clinical and administrative duties.

The position of ADON does not require an advanced degree. The ADON must have completed at least an associate's degree as an RN and must pass the licensure examination. As with the DON position, this person usually has had experience as an RN in the health-care setting, as well as some experience in a supervisory role.

ADONs will usually spend the majority of time completing administrative tasks; they are also responsible for providing direct patient care on an as-needed basis, especially in the absence of other nurses or nursing assistants.

The Nursing Home Reform Act (NHRA) mandates that Medicare- and Medicaid-certified nursing homes must have a DON and an RN on duty at least eight hours a day. In SNFs of sixty beds or less, the DON may also serve as the RN on duty.

REGISTERED NURSES

RNs are required to have at least an associate's degree or bachelor of science degree in nursing. A caveat to this requirement would be nurses from foreign countries who may have a different diploma or nurses who were graduates of the older-style, hospital-based nursing programs.

All skilled nursing facilities have an RN who is responsible for the direct care of patients and residents and is expected to have clinical nursing knowledge and possess teaching and procedural skills. RNs are not only responsible for conducting full body (head-to-toe) physical assessments but also for planning, providing, and documenting care according to physicians' orders.

RNs draw conclusions regarding diagnosis and are essentially the leaders of the health-care team. They are the only ones who can insert or manage a Foley catheter, touch or dress a percutaneous intravenous central catheter (PICC) line, start an IV, initiate certain treatments, or treat advanced wounds. Their role communicating with the patient or resident's doctor is crucial in the individual's health and well-being, including making judgments about when the doctor's immediate intervention is required.

Registered nurses are direct overseers of LPNs and CNAs and are responsible for implementing, coordinating, and supervising the care they provide. However, as per current law, regardless of the size of the skilled-nursing facility or nursing home, an RN is only required to be on duty eight hours a day.

At the time of this writing, the American Nurses Association (ANA) is asking for cosponsors of the Put a Registered Nurse in the Nursing Home Act (H.R.952) that would require SNFs and NHs that receive Medicare and Medicaid reimbursement to have at least one direct-care RN in the building at all times, even one serving in an administrative capacity. The bill was introduced by US Representative Jan Schakowsky on July 31, 2016. However, I have seen facilities where the evening supervisor is the only RN in buildings ranging from one hundred to three hundred beds. RNs in this situation have to oversee all clinical, administrative, and emergency situations, as well as conduct admission assessments.

While this may technically be consistent with present law, it creates an unsafe environment for patients or residents and staff. It would be preferable to have direct care RNs in the building, in addition to the supervising RN. It has become the modus operandi in many facilities to have a unit manager on the day shift as the only RN in charge of several units that are attended only by LPNs.

As discussed previously understaffing may increase the bottom line, but it is not in the best interest of patients. There have been numerous studies and articles that correlate staffing ratios with quality of care. One article links insufficient staffing to neglect and abuse, incidences of pressure ulcers, frequency of urinary tract infections, and the number of deficiency citations given.[84] It is disappointing that to date there are no national mandatory staffing ratios set forth by any regulatory agency for nursing homes and rehabilitation centers.

In an attempt to address improved nurse staffing, the government found that it fared no better when reimbursement was increased. Congress increased the nurse staffing component of SNF rates by 16.66 percent, effective April 1, 2001, raising rates for SNFs by 4 to 12 percent. Although the additional reimbursement focused on staff, the GAO found that SNFs' average nurse staffing increased by only 1.9 minutes per patient day, which did not equate to the increase in reimbursement rate.[85]

---

84 H. Y. Lee, M. A. Blegen, and C. Harrington, "The Effects of RN Staffing Hours on Nursing Home Quality: A Two-Stage Model," *International Journal of Nursing Studies* 51, no. 3 (2014): 409–17.

85 "Skilled Nursing Facilities: Available Data Show Average Nursing Staff Time Changed Little after Medicare Payment Increase," US Government Accountability Office, accessed June 2017, http://www.gao.gov/new.items/d03176.pdf.

LICENSED PRACTICAL NURSE (OR LICENSED VOCATIONAL NURSE [LVN] IN CALIFORNIA AND TEXAS)

An LPN works directly under the supervision of an RN. Educationally speaking, LPNs can earn a degree in twelve months or less as a practical nurse or receive a certificate of completion when coursework is completed through a technical-training school. This is very different from the professional nursing degree that is required for the registered nurse. Furthermore, while LPNs can dispense medication, take vital signs, give an injection, and do simple wound care, they cannot complete a full-body assessment or provide certain treatments (e.g., administering the first treatment for specific medications or starting an IV—unless they receive specific training to do so—and touch a PICC line).

There are some who refer to LPNs or LVNs derogatorily as "medication nurses" because they are often seen doing little more than dispensing medications. Because the salary for an LPN or LVN is understandably significantly less than for an RN, many facilities attempt to run with as few RNs in the building as possible (and, beyond the basic, eight-hour day shift, with none at all).

CERTIFIED NURSING ASSISTANT

A CNA is the one who performs the majority of the custodial ADLs for the patient or resident. This involves dressing, bathing, feeding assistance, and help in and out of bed. According to a 2016 PHI report, there are more than six hundred thousand nursing assistants who provide personal care, assistance with ADLs, and some measure of psychological, emotional, and clinical support to the estimated 1.4 million individuals who reside in the nation's nursing homes.[86] However, nursing assistants are generally not required to have a high school diploma or any prior work experience, and they receive minimum training and low wages, despite the fact that they perform some of the most physically demanding and challenging work in the facility.

According to OBRA '87 only a minimum amount of training is required to become a CNA (only seventy-five hours); the act does not establish mandates for a minimum staffing-to-patient ratio. The 2006 report from the American Association of Retired Persons (AARP) Public Policy Institute states that CNAs constitute 67 percent of the total nursing staff in nursing homes and that approximately 80 to 90 percent of a resident's interaction in the nursing home is with a CNA.[87] This is substantially higher than any other professional in a skilled-nursing facility. They have the most contact hours with patients and residents, providing the most hours of care, yet they are paid less than either RNs or LPNs and receive the least amount of training. That is because their job, seen as involving primarily custodial tasks (e.g., eating,

---

86 "US Nursing Assistants Employed in Nursing Homes: Key Facts," PHI, accessed September 2016, https://phinational.org/sites/default/files/phi-nursing-assistants-key-facts.pdf.

87 E. Hernandez-Medina, S. Eton, and D. Hurd, "Training Programs for Certified Nursing Assistants," AARP Public Policy Institute, accessed July 2017, https://assets.aarp.org/rgcenter/il/2006_08_cna.pdf.

bathing, dressing, toileting), is perceived as requiring the least amount of expertise. However, the observations made by a nurse aide regarding their patient or resident's physical, emotional, and cognitive status and slight changes thereof that are reportable to their nursing superiors—as well as knowledge of resident habits, likes and dislikes, and often-times familiarity with family members—far exceed any other professional in the nursing-home facility.

It is also worth mentioning that there are no federal requirements regarding the CNA's English literacy skills. There are some training programs that require the student to pass a reading and writing exam prior to enrolling in the training program. To effectively complete the job, which includes documenting the resident's daily habits and functioning, a CNA must have sufficient English reading and writing skills. However, in order to deliver quality care, the CNA must also be sufficiently fluent in order to understand directions and communicate with the majority of residents in their care. This has become a topic in our multicultural country, where many immigrants may seek a CNA position as entry-level employment. It also may be more accurate in particular areas of the country. However, the issue of communicating with patients and residents is a two-way street. Understanding residents who are nonnative English speakers or who may not speak the language at all is as big of a challenge as understanding the staff member whose first language is one other than English.

CNAs' patient workload continues to climb as cost-saving measures and profits are prioritized, resulting in shrinking time constraints per resident. Many of these aides are caring people who find a way to support, encourage, and meet resident needs in the most caring ways. However, there are many instances to the contrary. The continuous emphasis on cost-saving measures that affect staffing ratios is a formula for increased stress and frustration, possibility of injury, and potential for shortened tempers—all of which negatively impact the care being delivered to a medically compromised, frail, and often confused population.

There have been studies that have addressed the specifics of the tolls staff shortages take on RNs, and these stresses are certainly applicable to LPNs and CNAs. The risk of the staff's musculoskeletal injuries (MSDs) is documented. In 2012 a study by the US Department of Labor's Bureau of Labor Statistics found that RNs had 11,610 incidents of MSDs resulting in lost days at work.[88]

In a study entitled "Overtime Work and Incident Coronary Heart Disease: The Whitehall II Prospective Cohort Study," it was found that working long shifts and overtime has a detrimental effect on nurses' cardiovascular health.[89] This means they experience a greater incidence of heart disease. Besides the effect on physical health, there is the issue of physical and emotional exhaustion, often referred to as burnout. The physical effects

---

88 "Nonfatal Occupational Injuries and Illnesses Requiring Days Away from Work, 2015," US Department of Labor Bureau of Labor Statistics, accessed April 2017, https://www.bls.gov/news.release/osh2.nr0.htm. [82] M. Virtanen et al., "Overtime Work and Incident Coronary Heart Disease: The Whitehall II Prospective Cohort Study," *European Heart Journal* 31, no. 14 (2010): 1737–44, accessed June 2017, http://www.hal.inserm.fr/inserm-00488827.

of burnout can be characterized by chronic fatigue, irritability, insomnia, headaches, back pain, weight gain, depression, and high blood pressure.

A study cited in the *Journal of the American Medical Association* found that each additional patient in excess of four for which a nurse is responsible increases the risk of burnout up to 23 percent, as well as causing a 15 percent decrease in job satisfaction.[90] According to a 2012 study conducted by J. P. Cimiotti et al., one-third of nurses score equal to or greater than twenty-seven on a scale of emotional exhaustion. This correlates to a medical standard of high burnout.[91]

The NHRA that was part of OBRA '87 stipulated that nursing homes provide sufficient staff and services so that each resident will receive quality care, allowing each of them to attain or maintain the highest practical level of physical, mental, and psychosocial well-being. The ambiguity of this statement leaves tremendous room for interpretation. Left to those whose primary focus is profit and expedience, there is no incentive to provide staffing beyond bare minimum levels, regardless of facility size.

There are, however, some positive developments in the area of staffing. A 2001 study by Harrington and Millman reported

---

90 "Safe-Staffing Ratios: Benefiting Nurses and Patients," Department for Professional Employees, accessed June 2017, http://dpeaflcio.org/programs-publications/issue-fact-sheets/safe-staffing-ratios-benefiting-nurses-and-patients.

91 J. P. Cimiotti, L. H. Aiken, D. M. Sloane, and E. S. Wu, "Nurse Staffing, Burnout, and Health-Care Associated Infection," *American Journal of Infection Control* 40, no. 6 (2012): 486–90. Accessed September 2017, doi:10.1016/j.ajic.2012.02.029.

that there were states that stipulated staffing requirements that exceeded the federal guidelines as follows:

- Fifteen states exceeded the staffing standards for RNs, and twenty-five states had higher standards for LPNs.
- Eight states required that facilities of one hundred beds or more must have an RN on duty twenty-four hours a day.
- Thirty-three states have minimum staffing requirements for CNAs.[92]

Due to the problems nursing shortages cause for the patient, the worker, and the system at large, there has been a growing number of states enacting legislation addressing this issue, albeit mostly as it relates to hospitals. As of December 2015, the following fourteen states have, either through legislation or regulations, established nursing staffing levels: California, Connecticut, Illinois, Massachusetts, Minnesota, Nevada, New Jersey, New York, Ohio, Oregon, Rhode Island, Texas, Vermont, and Washington.

Seven additional states now require hospitals to have committees dedicated to staffing policy (Connecticut, Illinois, Nevada, Ohio, Oregon, Texas, and Washington). Five additional states have moved to full disclosure or requisite public reporting of

---

92 C. Harrington and M. Millman, "Survey of State Staffing Standards Included in a Report Prepared for the Henry J. Kaiser Family Foundation," University of California, San Francisco, accessed April 2017, https://books.google.com/books?isbn=0763707538.

staffing (Illinois, New Jersey, New York, Rhode Island, and Vermont).

As of September 2015, sixteen states now prohibit mandated overtime for nurses, except in the event of a public health emergency (Arkansas, California, Connecticut, Illinois, Maryland, Minnesota, Missouri, New Jersey, New Hampshire, New York, Oregon, Pennsylvania, Rhode Island, Texas, Washington, and West Virginia).

I have seen many facilities strong-arm nurses into overtime. Many succumb to the pressure as a sense of duty and responsibility to their patients and colleagues, as well as the fear of job loss. The reason for the shortage of available nurses in many cases stems from the low wages paid from large, for-profit corporations whose motive appears to be to get the most for less. Nurses who have the flexibility can pick and choose to work for hospitals or facilities that will pay them fair wages for their professional expertise.

The ANA attempted—but failed—to provide nurses the opportunity to have an integral role in formulating national standards for nursing staffing levels during the session of the 113th Congress (2014–2015). The Registered Nurse Safe Staffing Act was introduced to the House of Representatives in 2015 and was not moved out of committee for a vote. This bill addressed hospitals that participate in Medicare-reimbursement plans.

US Representative Barbara Boxer introduced the National Nursing Shortage Reform and Patient Advocacy Act in March 2015, which would establish specific nurse-to-patient ratios for hospitals and other facilities. US Representative Jan Schakowsky reintroduced the Nursing Staffing Standards for Patient Safety and Quality Care Act of 2015, the purpose of which was to establish federal standards for nursing-to-patient ratios for all hospitals nationwide. It would also provide a national standard disallowing nursing overtime, except in strict cases of emergency. This legislation has been endorsed by the American Federation of Labor and Congress of Industrial Organizations (AFL-CIO), the American Federation of Government Employees (AFGE), the American Federation of Teachers (AFT), National Nurses United (NNU), and the United Steelworkers (USW). There is no information to date as to whether the bill ever made it out of committee for a vote. However, considering the fate of other legislative efforts and rulings that have been overturned seemingly reflecting more accommodations to owners and providers, it seems doubtful that the efforts that would benefit individuals but possibly impact costs and profit to owners or providers will succeed.

It is hopeful that the requirements set forth by ACA regarding staff reporting and the subsequent Payroll-Based Journal established by CMS, may be a step towards establishing minimum nursing standards in skilled nursing facilities.

REHABILITATION DEPARTMENT

REHABILITATION STAFF

This department is headed by a director who, under most circumstances, is either a physical or occupational therapist. The director oversees the therapy caseloads and structures therapy minutes, based on therapists' assessments and recommendations as well as on the individual's type of insurance. As stated previously Medicare Part A patients usually receive the most therapy-intervention minutes across the most therapy days in the week. The department consists of a variety of therapists:

PHYSICAL THERAPIST (MAY ALSO BE DOCTORS OF PHYSICAL THERAPY [DPT])

The PT evaluates all residents and develops a plan of care based on the results of the evaluation. They are required to have at least a master's degree. Some schools now offer a doctor of physical therapy (DPT) degree, which has more of a medical-based curriculum. Though some DPTs refer to themselves as doctors, they should not be confused with medical doctors, as they do not attend medical school.

PHYSICAL THERAPY ASSISTANTS

Physical therapy assistants (PTAs) are often the therapists who treat the patient or resident, although—depending on the case load—the physical therapist may treat as well. PTAs cannot legally treat any patient or resident unless a PT is present in the building. They are also not permitted to complete evaluations. They may have either four years of college or a two-year associate's degree plus two years of training. The notes they write are required to be countersigned and approved by the physical therapist in charge.

OCCUPATIONAL THERAPIST

The lead occupational therapist may be referred to as a registered occupational therapist (OTR) and must hold a master's degree. OTRs evaluate patients or residents and develop the treatment plan, but they may also treat, depending on staffing and caseload. They must countersign the notes for all certified occupational therapy assistants (COTAs).

OCCUPATIONAL THERAPY ASSISTANTS (CERTIFIED OCCUPATIONAL THERAPY ASSISTANTS OR OCCUPATIONAL THERAPY ASSISTANTS)

COTAs are more often than not the treating therapists. They cannot perform evaluations, but they can treat patients or residents without having an OTR in the building. They have two years of training beyond either four years of college or an associate's degree.

SPEECH THERAPIST OR SPEECH-LANGUAGE PATHOLOGIST

Speech and language pathologists (STs or SLPs) must have a master's degree and are responsible for evaluating, developing the plan of care, and treating patients or residents in the areas of speech, language, communication, and swallowing. They determine appropriate solid and liquid food consistencies to ensure patients or residents can swallow safely.

SOCIAL WORKERS

Social workers serve as the liaison between the patients or residents, loved ones, and staff and are responsible for providing psychosocial support. They also usually take the lead role in care-plan meetings. The social worker is responsible for coordinating discharge planning, whether from a hospital to a nursing home or rehabilitation facility or from a facility to the community at large.

When a patient is admitted to a facility, the social worker usually completes a Brief Interview of Mental Status (BIMS) assessment, which serves as a snapshot of the individual's cognitive functioning and is a tool used as an indicator of dementia. It should be noted that a patient can achieve a high score on the BIMS and be alert and oriented to person, place, and time (known as "oriented times three"), but the individual can still present with poor decision-making ability. The social worker should be able to get a sense of the individual's ability in that area during the assessment session. Ideally the BIMS should be administered on a quarterly basis for determining any change in cognitive status—whether an improvement or a decline.

Another assessment tool administered by the social worker is known as the Patient Health Questionnaire (PHQ-9), which is a series of questions used to determine if the individual is depressed.

The skilled-nursing facility is based on a medical model; patients and residents in these facilities also have psychosocial, mental health, and quality-of-life needs. They often experience feelings of loneliness, boredom, and depression associated with loss of control and independence. Though facilities usually have consulting psychologists and psychiatrists, the social worker is probably the only full-time qualified staff member, by training and experience, who can evaluate and provide psychosocial and mental health support.

Because of the number of patients for whom they are responsible (ranging up to 120 patients, according to the New York State Department of Health), as well as the scope and extent of their duties and responsibilities regarding admissions, care plan, and other special-request meetings; explaining insurance (whether it be Medicare or Medicaid eligibility) and its requisite forms and paperwork; discharging patients; and addressing the myriad facility patient/resident issues that may arise, social workers may have little time to address these vital mental-health issues.

As per OBRA '87, federal guidelines for SNFs of up to 120 beds do not require a qualified social worker on staff, but facilities are required to provide psychosocial and mental health services. There are states that have adopted stricter standards than those set forth by the federal government as it pertains to social worker availability within SNFs.

According to the National Association of Social Workers (NASW), there are several levels of social workers who can be found in a skilled-nursing facility. They are listed below, with their respective educational requirements.[93]

1. Licensed clinical social workers who have a degree at the master's level or above
2. Consulting social workers who may or may not provide direct services to patients or residents. They may also supervise social-work staff as needed (i.e., bachelor's-level staff).
3. Social workers who hold a bachelor's level degree
4. Social-work designees who may hold a bachelor's degree but in a field other than social work
5. Those without any degree but who may have been grandfathered in as a social-work designee

There are also circumstances in which an individual may not have a specific degree in social work but has sufficient, related-degree coursework. I have a colleague who holds a master's degree in gerontology/administration and a certificate in long-term-care administration. Her position on the short-term rehabilitation unit of a nursing home and rehabilitation center was that of a full-fledged social worker and included the same duties and responsibilities as for one who holds a master's degree in social work.

---

93 J. O'Neill and A. L. Rosen, *Professional Social Work Services in Skilled Nursing Facilities: Survey of Current Practices and Recommendations* July 1998 National Association of Social Workers, Washington, D.C. September 9, 2017

DIETITIAN

Most facilities have a registered dietitian who is responsible for ensuring that the kitchen staff accurately fulfills the therapeutic diet ordered by an individual's doctor. The dietitian and speech pathologist should work closely to ensure that the kitchen accurately delivers any modified solid or liquid diet consistencies based on patient or resident need and as recommended by the speech pathologist and physician.

Shortly after admission the dietitian usually meets with the patient or resident and/or family regarding the person's food preferences, likes and dislikes, and food allergies. The dietitian is also responsible for educating the family and patient or resident about particular dietary needs while in the facility, as well as upon discharge. In the event the patient receives tube feedings, the dietitian will also work closely with nursing and the medical doctor to determine the appropriate calories, formula, and manner of administration. Family members and patients should feel free to ask questions about any issues or concerns about alternative forms of feeding.

NURSING HOME ADMINISTRATOR

Nursing-home administrators must hold at least a bachelor's degree, although many also hold a master's degree in health administration or a related area (e.g., long-term-care administration, health-services administration, public-health administration, or business administration). The degree must include courses in long-term care/health care, gerontology, and personnel management. If one holds a bachelor's degree, only fifteen credit hours of requisite courses are needed in those related areas.

The educational programs for administrators also include coursework in building operations, business and leadership, marketing, organizational behavior, health-care law, regulations, and ethics, as well as information systems and medical statistics. In every state, including the District of Columbia, administrators must complete a state-approved training program as well as an internship and pass the licensure examination.

The Commission on Accreditation of Healthcare Management Education (CAHME) is responsible for accreditation of the professional degrees in health-care management that facility administrators receive. The organization has a website that lists all qualifying programs by state.

The primary daily responsibilities of the administrator are related to decisions regarding admitting patients, managing overall building operations, managing staff, budgeting, accounting, and financial planning. The administrator's responsibilities include:

* Ensuring that the facility is in compliance with the state and federal health and safety codes
* Preparing official reports regarding the status of the facility
* Setting facility goals and coordinating programs within the facility
* Ultimate responsibility for the financial success of the facility

• • •

Staffing Incongruity or Staffing Misapplied

The facility in which I worked admitted a female patient in her fifties who had significant psychological and behavioral issues without any other significant impairments. She was alert, verbal and totally physically able-bodied (or PA). This facility had only recently been purchased by a corporate entity that owned approximately forty facilities. The corporation wasted no time in cutting costs. Within a matter of weeks there were staff shortages on all units, and direct care costs were visibly reduced, from availability of basic daily supplies for resident care to the food quality, amount of food, and food choices provided. The staff was frustrated and tired. Why is this important? Because this female patient walked independently and rode the elevators from floor to floor, there was concern she would cause harm to herself or to others or that she could wander out of the facility, with the potential for serious consequences.

The solution was one-to-one supervision throughout the day. All levels of personnel were hired on their off days to accompany the resident every minute of every day for several weeks. From CNAs to kitchen staff, someone accompanied the resident every waking moment of the day, no matter where she went.

The incongruity of the situation seemed ridiculous. The new ownership was cutting costs down to bare-bones levels. Ownership even went so far as to lengthen the time period between staff paychecks as a maneuver to either avoid paying staff or frustrate long-time staff members with higher pay and greater benefits so they would leave, (After a couple of months this was found to be illegal and had to be reversed). Yet the resident continued to reside in the facility, and administration continued to authorize paying for the one-to-one supervision. The money spent on that resident could easily have been spent on adding a CNA or a nurse to any shift on any floor that was short staffed to avoid staff members feeling strained and stretched to care for the residents.

The situation went on for approximately several weeks before the resident was transferred out of the facility.

Dignity versus Staffing

I met a colleague from the South-Central state in which a New York based company recently purchased over a dozen facilities. My colleague recounted that she was familiar with one of those facilities where residents were already complaining about the decline in food quality. Furthermore, she reported that the pull-up undergarments have gotten noticeably thinner and staff has begun having residents where two at a time. The reason was not only to avoid inadvertent leakage due to the thinner garments, but also because fewer staff hours would be needed to change people more frequently.

Physiologic Need versus Staffing

I work in a facility in which a patient's family member who is also an RN recounted the following situation. During one of her visits she encountered a resident calling out to go to the bathroom. She informed the resident she could not assist him but would locate a staff member. She walked up and down the corridor of the unit finally coming upon a CNA after several minutes. She told the CNA of the resident's need and was shocked by the reply: "we only take residents to the bathroom twice a day; there isn't enough staff to do it more often." She insisted the CNA attend to the resident or she would report her. (of course, thinking of her own mother in this same situation) She felt the staff member was rude and appeared impatient with the resident so she remained close by the resident's room to hear what transpired once the CNA and the resident were inside. She said the CNA repeatedly asked the resident while he was using the bathroom in what seemed to be an indignant voice, "are you finished?"

This same facility had been recently purchased by a for-profit corporation that owned approximately Forty facilities.

CHAPTER 9

Bundled-Payment System: An Alternative Reimbursement Method

• • •

BUNDLED PAYMENTS ARE KNOWN BY a variety of other names: episode-based payment, episodic payment, episode-of-care payment, evidence-based case rate, global bundled payment, global package, or packaged pricing to name a few. It is a reimbursement system where health-care providers (whether hospitals, physicians, or nursing homes) are paid one fee based on a particular clinical episode. Bundled payments have long been proposed as a means of reducing health-care costs and were integral to the debate on health-care reform in the United States during President Obama's administration. Commercial insurance providers have been proponents of the bundled-payment system as a means of cost reduction. As of 2012 there are estimates that a substantial percentage (possibly as high as 33 percent) of health-care reimbursement in the United States used some form of a bundled-payment methodology.

As early as the mid-1980s, it was thought that hospitals were prematurely discharging patients to skilled nursing facilities in an effort to save money. The proposed solution was a bundled-payment system whereby Medicare would pay one fee for an inpatient hospital stay and post hospital stay for the same clinical episode. Though the proposed bundled-payment system had many proponents, as of 2009 there was not widespread implementation.

Research shows that as early as 1984 there were isolated attempts to use the bundled-payment system. It was the Texas Heart Institute that began to charge flat fees for both hospital and physician services for cardiovascular surgeries. It claimed that this approach maintained a high quality of care while lowering costs. (In 1985 the flat fee for coronary artery bypass surgery at the Institute was $13,800, versus the average Medicare payment of $24,588.)[94]

There were other attempts to use the system between 1987 and 1989. In one experiment at Ingham Regional Medical Center in Michigan, the hospital's orthopedic surgeon developed a scenario in which the HMO referred 111 patients to the surgeon for possible surgery.[95] Patients were not charged a fee for the evaluation, but in the event surgery was recommended, the surgeon and hospital received a one-time predetermined fee for any arthroscopic surgery performed. In addition, a two-year warranty was provided, which indicated that the facility would assume financial responsibility for any post-surgery expenses and up to four repeat operations for the same condition if needed.

This arrangement seemed to benefit all parties involved. Results indicated that the HMO paid $193,000 instead of the $318,538 expected; the hospital received $96,500, rather than the $84,892 expected; and the surgeon and his associates received $96,500, instead of the $51,877 expected.

---

94 C. Edmonds and G. L. Hallman, "Cardiovascular Care Providers: A Pioneer in Bundled Services, Shared Risk, and Single Payment," *Texas Heart Institute Journal* 22, no. 1 (1995): 72–76. Accessed May 2017 https://www.ncbi.nlm.nih.gov/pmc/articles/PMC325213/

95 L. L. Johnson and R. L. Becker, "An Alternative Health-Care Reimbursement System—Application of Arthroscopy and Financial Warranty: Results of a Two-year Pilot Study," *Arthroscopy* 10, no. 4 (1994): 462–70, discussion 471–72, accessed May 2017, http://bostonshoulderinstitute.com/wp-content/uploads/2015/03/Johnson-et-al-1987-An-Alternative-Healthcare-Reimbursement-System-Arthroscopy-and-Financial-Warranty.pdf.

There was a follow-up to this study in 1991 when a Medicare Participating Heart-Bypass Center Demonstration was initiated in four hospitals across the United States.[96] In 1993 there were three additional hospitals added to the project before it came to conclusion in 1996. Essentially Medicare paid hospitals one global rate for inpatient hospital and physician fees for coronary artery bypass surgical hospitalizations as well as for readmissions related to the same condition. Published evaluations of the project concluded the following:

1. One analysis in 1997 found that between 1991 and 1993 the original four hospitals in the demonstration saved approximately $15.31 million for Medicare and $1.84 million for Medicare beneficiaries and supplemental insurance carriers under the global-payment system (a total savings of $17.2 million). The original expected Medicare payment was $110.8 million for coronary artery bypass surgeries. In addition, it was determined that there was no reduction in the quality of care provided and that of the total savings, 85 to 93 percent could be attributed to the inpatient stay while 6 to 11 percent could

---

96 J. Cromwell et al., "Medicare Participating Heart Bypass Demonstration," Centers for Medicare & Medicaid Services, accessed April 2017, https://www.cms.gov/Research-Statistics-Data-and-Systems/Statistics-Trends-and-Reports/Reports/downloads/oregon2_1998_3.pdf, hereafter cited as "Medicare Participating Heart Bypass Demonstration").

be attributed to the care following the patient's discharge from the hospital.[97]

2. A 1998 report to the Health Care Financing Administration (since renamed CMS) concluded that the total savings for the seven hospitals studied in the five years of the demonstration project equaled $42.3 million for Medicare and $7.9 for Medicare beneficiaries and their supplemental insurance carriers. In addition, even taking into account patient risk factors, the inpatient mortality rate in the demonstration hospitals declined over the course of the project. Negative aspects of the project were difficulties in billing and collection.[98]

3. A 2001 paper examined the micro-costs at three of the original four hospitals and found that "the cost reductions primarily came from nursing intensive care unit, routine nursing, pharmacy, and catheter lab."[99]

---

97 J. Cromwell, D. A. Dayhoff, and A. H. Thoumaian, "Cost Savings and Physician Responses to Global Bundled Payments for Medicare Heart Bypass Surgery," *Health Care Financing Review* 19, no. 1 (1997): 41–57, accessed February 2017, https://www.ncbi.nlm.nih.gov/pubmed/10180001.

98 "Medicare Participating Heart Bypass Demonstration."

99 C. F. Liu, S. Subramanian, and J. Cromwell, "Impact of Global Bundled Payments on Hospital Costs of Coronary Artery Bypass Grafting," Journal of Health Care Finance 27, no. 4 (2001): 39–54, accessed March 2017, https://iths.pure.elsevier.com/.../impact-of-global-bundled-payments-on-hospital-costs-of-coronary-artery-bypass-grafting.

By 2001 what was referred to as "case rates for episodes of illness" (i.e., bundled payments) were regarded as a kind of blended payment method, taking into account the following:

1. The retrospective payment system where bills are submitted to services after they are performed
2. The prospective payment system in which a set fee is established and paid based on projected provided services
3. Fee-for-service system where bills are submitted separately for each service provided in real time
4. Capitation with a ceiling for billable fees—sometimes combined with fee-for-service or bills for specialty services or budgets[100]

These plans also consider what is known as "comprehensive payment for comprehensive care"[101] and complete chronic care, which takes into account payments for wellness care (preventive medicine). The plans attempt to maintain health and wellness but allow for specific episodes of illness.

With passing years there were additional demonstration projects that tested the bundled-payment system. In 2003 the St. Joseph Hospital in Denver, Colorado, conducted a demonstration project for an acute-care episode (ACE) that was

---

100 D. J. Satin and J. Miles, "Performance-Based Bundled Payments: Potential Benefits and Burdens," *Minnesota Medicine* 92, no. 10 (2009): 33–35.

101 A. H. Goroll, R. A. Berenson, S. C. Schoenbaum, and L. B. Gardner, "Fundamental Reform of Payment for Adult Primary Care: Comprehensive Payment for Comprehensive Care," *Journal of General Internal Medicine* 22, no. 3 (2007): 410–15. accessed March 2017, https://www.ncbi.nlm.nih.gov/pmc/articles/PMC1824766/

based on the Medicare Prescription Drug Improvement and Modernization Act. The project essentially bundled Medicare Parts A and B for what was known as specific-care episodes.

In 2006 to 2007 there was once again a project testing coronary artery bypass surgery practices—known as the Geisinger Health System. The system tested a "ProvenCare" model that was conducted by the Geisinger Health System. The project focused on best practices from the initial stages, when the patient first presented to the health-care professional, to preoperative, inpatient, and postoperative care. In addition, it examined incidences of rehospitalizations within ninety days of discharge "packaged into a fixed price."[102]

This project was nationally acclaimed and reported by both the *New York Times* and the *New England Journal of Medicine*.[103] A 2007 evaluation of the project found results similar to past projects: 117 patients who received ProvenCare had a significantly shorter total length of stay (resulting in 5 percent lower hospital charges, a greater likelihood of being discharged to home, and a lower readmission rate compared with 137 patients who received conventional care in 2005).[104]

---

102 A. S. Casale et al., "'ProvenCare[SM]': A Provider-Driven Pay-for-Performance Program for Acute Episodic Cardiac Surgical Care," *Annals of Surgery* 246, no. 4 (2007): 613–21, discussion 621–23, accessed February 2017, https://www.ncbi.nlm.nih.gov/pubmed/17893498, (hereafter cited as "'ProvenCare[SM]': A Provider-Driven Pay-for-Performance Program for Acute Episodic Cardiac Surgical Care").

103 T. H. Lee, "Pay for Performance, Version 2.0?" *New England Journal of Medicine* 357, no. 6 (2007): 531–33, accessed May 2017, www.nejm.org/doi/full/10.1056/NEJMp078124.

104 "'ProvenCare[SM]': A Provider-Driven Pay-for-Performance Program for Acute Episodic Cardiac Surgical Care."

Medicare officials, as well as others at the top of the health industry, took a keen interest in Geisinger's ProvenCare program. In 2008 there were proposed expansions to include other episodes of care: hip replacement surgery, cataract surgery, percutaneous coronary intervention, bariatric surgery, lower-back surgery, and perinatal care. Geisinger's project continued to receive acclaim in 2009 as the news media reported on it as a model for health-care reform to be proposed by President Obama.[105]

Beginning in 2007 grants were offered by the Robert Wood Johnson Foundation to further examine the efficacy of a bundled-payment system. The project was called Provider Payment Reform for Outcomes, Margins, Evidence, Transparency, Hassle-reduction, Excellence, Understandability, and Sustainability (PROMETHEUS) Payment. It was conducted for the purpose of developing "evidence-informed case rates."[106] These rates took into account, and were adjusted for, the severe or complex nature of a patient's illness, based on the documentation or evidence provided by the health-care practitioner (thus the name evidence-informed case rates).

In this method of service delivery, health-care providers would receive a bonus if their quarterly spending came in under budget. In the event their spending was over budget, their

---

105 C. Connolly, "For This Health System, Less Is More. Program That Guarantees Doing Things Right the First Time, for Flat Fee, Pays Off," *Washington Post*, March 31, 2009. HIghBeam Research accessed September 2017, https://www.highbeam.com/publications/the-washington-post-p5554/mar-31-2009

106 A. G. Gosfield, "Making PROMETHEUS Payment Rates Real: Ya' Gotta Start Somewhere," Robert Wood Johnson Foundation, last modified June 2008, accessed June 2017, www.rwjf.org/en/library/research/2009/06/what-is-prometheus-payment-.html.

payment would be withheld pending a review. There were three pilot sites for this project, which ended in 2011.

By mid-2008 the MedPAC made a concerted effort to find a way to use a bundled-payment system. One method that was recommended was for the secretary of health and human services to examine what was known as a virtual bundling. With this method health-care providers would receive separate payments; they could also be given financial rewards or be penalized based on their levels of spending. A pilot program would be established "to test the feasibility of actual bundled payment for services around hospitalization episodes for select conditions."[107]

However, prior to the release of that report, the CMS announced that it was conducting a Medicare Acute Care Episode (ACE) demonstration project for bundling payments for certain cardiovascular and orthopedic procedures. The bundling payments for this project were limited to in-hospital and physician charges and did not include post-hospitalization care. There were five project location sites in four states that carried out the project: Colorado, New Mexico, Oklahoma, and Texas. In this project Medicare was given discounts of 1 to 6 percent for the selected procedures, and Medicare beneficiaries received a financial incentive ranging anywhere from $250 to $1,157 to have a procedure done in one of the demonstration hospitals.

Interest in bundled payments continued in the US Senate and were the subject of a white paper by Senator Max Baucus,

---

107 "Chapter 4: A Path to Bundled Payment around a Hospitalization," Medicare Payment Advisory Commission, June 2008 accessed February 2017, 67.59.137.244/chapters/Jun08_Ch04.pdf.

chair of the Senate Finance Committee in November 2008. The white paper recommended that the Medicare ACE demonstration expand to other sites, focus on other clinical conditions if certain criteria were met, and include services that were provided post-hospitalization.[108]

The Special Commission on the Health Care Payment System in Massachusetts, in July of 2009, distinguished between episode-based payments (or bundled payments) and global payments (which are fixed-dollar payment amounts for the care that patients may receive in a given time period). The commission thought the episode-based (or bundled-payment) system placed a financial risk on health-care providers as it related both to the occurrence of medical conditions and the management of those conditions. The commission recommended that the global-payment system was preferable for health-care providers in that state and that it should include financial incentives as a reward for accessible and high-quality care. The commission also believed the global-payment system had a greater potential to reduce episodes of care, and the state had a positive prior experience with this payment system.

The Lewin Group, a health-care consulting firm, published a report for the CMS in which it analyzed sixty thousand episodes of care between October 2013 and September 2014 by 130 hospitals, sixty-three skilled nursing facilities, and four physician-group practices that participated in three of the four

---

108 M. Baucus, "Call to Action," American Health Lawyers Association, accessed February 2017, https://www.healthlawyers.org/Members/PracticeGroups/TaskForces/HRE/Documents/CalltoAction_HealthcareReform.pdf.

bundled-payment-for-care-improvement programs. The report did not fully endorse the bundled-payment system as being an effective payment model for several reasons: the size and time frame of the sample were insufficient for drawing conclusions about the system's efficacy, and the duration that the system had been used was insufficient.

As of 2010 the Patient Protection and Affordable Care Act and the Affordable Health Care for America Act included provisions for incorporating bundled payments and called for a national Medicare pilot program starting in 2013, with possible expansion into 2016. The bill required "a plan to reform Medicare payments for postacute services, including bundled payments."[109] The CMS spearheaded an initiative in which 450 health-care organizations participated in what was known as Bundled Payments for Care Improvement (BPCI). The purpose of the initiative was to determine if bundling payments for services was a viable method for improving quality of care and lowering costs. In June 2016 CMS announced it would extend the program for two more years.

The CMS announced a proposal for its new ninety-day bundled payment program in July 2015. It mandated that the ninety-day bundled payment model be applied to Medicare beneficiaries who undergo joint replacement; this is also known as the Comprehensive Care for Joint Replacement Initiative. It is based on the 2011 BPCI program as a well as research from

---

109 "Side-by-Side Comparison of Major Health Care Reform Proposals," Henry J. Kaiser Family Foundation, accessed April 2017,_http://www.kff.org/health-reform/issue-brief/side-by-side-comparison-of-major-health-care-reform-proposals/.

the ACE demonstration project. It is expected that this new program will have a favorable impact on cost efficiency, quality of care, patient outcomes, and collaboration among providers for an episode of care, as well as eliminating unnecessary testing and treatments.

In July 2016 CMS announced three new bundles, referred to as episode-payment models (EPMs), aimed at cardiovascular-care procedures including acute myocardial infarction (AMI) or heart attack, coronary artery bypass graft (CABG) or bypass surgery, and hip/femur fractures. The new model went into effect on July 1, 2017.

Some of the advantages of the bundled payment system have been discussed in the history of its development. However, there are additional pros and cons that are worthy of consideration.

PROS

It is a widely held belief by both payment providers and the population at large that approximately 25 to 30 percent of hospital procedures are unnecessary and do not improve quality of care. Because a bundled payment is a lump-sum payment per episodic condition, it may be a disincentive to providing, and thus billing for, unnecessary care. Furthermore, there is a likelihood that this system encourages greater coordination and communication among providers, which would translate into improving quality of care.

Bundled payment, because it is calculated based on an individual episode of care or condition, does not seem to penalize or provide a disincentive to health-care providers for caring for sicker patients.

Considering the advantages and disadvantages of other payment methods (e.g., fee-for-service, pay-for-performance, and global payment such as capitation), some researchers determined that "episode payments are the most immediately viable approach."[110]

The Rand Corporation enlisted researchers who determined an estimate of 5.4 percent reduction in health-care spending between 2010 and 2019 if the PROMETHEUS model for bundled payment for selected conditions and procedures was widely used.[111] The corporation determined that the savings using the bundled-payment system was significantly higher than for seven other possible methods for reducing national health expenditures. In addition, Rand found that bundled payments would decrease financial risk to consumers and would decrease waste.[112]

❋ Bundling payment can reduce inefficiency and duplication of services, as well as unnecessary care, and it eliminates the failure to provide appropriate postoperative care.

---

110 R. E. Mechanic and S. H. Altman, "Payment Reform Options: Episode Payment Is a Good Place to Start," *Health Affairs* 28, no. 2 (2009): 262–71, accessed May 2017, content. healthaffairs.org/content/28/2/w262.full.pdf+html.

111 P. S. Hussey, C. Eibner, M. S. Ridgely, and E. A. McGlynn, "Controlling US Health Care Spending—Separating Promising from Unpromising Approaches," *New England Journal of Medicine* 361, no. 22 (2009): 2109–11, accessed June 2017, https://www.ncbi. nlm.nih.gov/pubmed/19907037.

112 "Analysis of Bundled Payment," RAND Corporation, accessed February 2017, https:// www.rand.org/pubs/technical_reports/TR562z20/analysis-of-bundled-payment.html.

* This method of payment is more transparent. Fixed prices for episodes of care and patient outcomes can be published and readily available for consumers to assist them in making informed choices about providers based on actual information.

* Bundled payments may also encourage larger hospitals or health-system networks to become more economical by negotiating better prices for purchasing in bulk if providers agree to use a particular product or type of medical supply.

Cons

* There is insufficient scientific evidence on bundled payments and the model's effect on health outcomes. Physicians could hospitalize patients for a condition that would not necessarily require hospitalization in order to overstate the severity of an illness or condition, escalating it to an "episode of care."

* Providers who may be less scrupulous and want to maximize profits may also provide lower levels of care, or the lowest level of care possible. They may intentionally overlook or not diagnose complications from treatment if they occur near the end of the bundled-payment period. They may also delay needed post-hospital care pending the end of the bundled-payment period, which could negatively impact a patient's overall condition. Hospitals

also, in an effort to maximize profits, could limit access to specialists or special treatments during an inpatient hospitalization.

* If a provider has to outsource part of a patient's care, as in the case of having the patient consult another specialist for a particular episodic condition, it may be difficult to determine financial accountability for a given bundled payment.

* There are administrative and operational complications in establishing fair compensation rates. Small sample sizes and incomplete data may cause difficulties in calculating proper rates for bundled payments. In the event rates are set too high, health-care providers may continue to provide unnecessary services; setting rates too low may result in patients receiving inadequate care, as well as cause financial hardship for the provider.

* A bundled-payment system may not be able to be applied to all illnesses across the board. There could be instances when a patient may have multiple care episodes that overlap each other, and the bundled payments would overlap, which could become cumbersome.

According to one article, "Academic health centers, which emphasize research, teaching, and new technologies, may be disadvantaged by the payment scheme."[113] Under the bundled-

---

113 A. Robinow, "The Potential of Global Payment: Insights from the Field," The Commonwealth Fund, accessed December 2016, http://www.commonwealthfund.org/~/media/Files/Publications/Fund%20Report/2010/Feb/1373_Robinow_potential_global_payment.pdf.

payment method, if a patient experiences a catastrophic illness or event, the health-care provider could potentially experience a large financial loss.

There is significant variation in the application of health care across the United States, primarily due to a lack of standardization in health-care protocols, as reported in a study by Dartmouth Medical School.[114] Currently there is no nationally accepted bundled-payment methodology, and we can expect continued experimentation with this model.

As patient's we place our trust in physicians and other health-care professionals to make the best medical decisions for our health and well-being. However, one can easily see that their decisions can be motivated by other factors, especially if the providers are profit-driven. When this is the case, the health-care industry does not necessarily serve our best medical interests and needs.

It seems prudent to do research on one's own particular condition, not for purposes of challenging the physician or questioning his or her medical expertise but to be armed with sufficient information to ask intelligent questions about the course of prescribed treatments, possible complications, and overall recommendations. In the event the answers do not seem to be consistent with one's own research, it may be the wisest practical decision to seek alternatives or at least a second opinion.

---

114 D. Baggot, "The Bundled Payment Title Wave: Recap and Insight from the Fourth National Bundled Payment Summit," Oregon Healthcare News, July 7, 2014, accessed August 2017, http://www.revolvy.com/main/index.php?s=Bundled%20 payment&item_type=topic.

The bundled-payment system is clearly not the only potential health-care change, and we must be vigilant and ask questions of those making decisions on our behalf.

The CMS issued a press release on August 15, 2015, effectively reducing the mandatory number of geographic areas participating in this model from sixty-seven to thirty-four and providing for the remaining thirty-three areas to participate on only a voluntary basis.[115] Furthermore it proposed canceling the Episodic Payment Model and the Cardiac Rehabilitation Incentive Payment model that was to be implemented on January 1, 2018. The explanation provided was that, by eliminating these models, the CMS would provide the liberty and flexibility for investigating, designing, and testing other options that would improve the quality and coordination of care during both the inpatient and postacute periods. Though the bundled-payment system was in its fledgling stages of application, considering the decades of successful research initiatives and pilot projects that went into the creating this model, one can only wonder the reasoning behind the cancellation of the model that has demonstrated to be effective in reining in the astronomical costs for CMS, patients, and insurance companies.

On a personal level, I know of SNF administrators, doctors, and owners who were not in favor of the model because of the capped reimbursement dollars for particular care episodes,

---

115 "CMS Proposes Changes to the Comprehensive Care for Joint Replacement Model, Cancellation of the Mandatory Episode Payment Models and Cardiac Rehabilitation Incentive Payment Model," Centers for Medicare & Medicaid Services, accessed November 2016, https://www.cms.gov/Newsroom/MediaReleaseDatabase/Factsheets/2017-Fact-Sheet-items/2017-08-15.html.

thereby affecting the types and numbers of admissions they would receive or be willing to accept, as well as the potential for alternative, post-acute rehabilitation services that could be provided. As reported in a previous chapter in which the CMA reported that CMS had already acknowledged that lobbying efforts affected its decision regarding willingness to adjust reimbursement rates despite evidence of overpayment in the hundreds of millions of dollars, it would lead one to conclude that similar efforts may have impacted this decision.

It remains to be seen when and what process or program in particular will be proposed as an alternative, cost-saving measure.

CHAPTER 10

New Trends in Nursing-Home Reform

• • •

Use of Medications to Control Behavior

This rather alert and verbal patient in her early seventies was admitted to a short-term rehabilitation unit after being hospitalized for the repair of a broken hip. On this particular morning E. H. had to use the bathroom before she began eating her breakfast, which had already been delivered to her room located just a few doors down from the nursing station. She rang for assistance, but after almost three-quarters of an hour, no one came to assist her with her toileting needs.

In a desperate attempt to get someone's attention, she picked up the tray from the bedside table on which it was placed and, with all her might, flung it into the doorway which was in direct line of her bed. This, of course, had the desired effect; nurses and nurse aides came running to the room to find out what had happened. The patient explained that she had been ringing for assistance to use the bathroom and no one came to assist her and, because she feared having an "accident" in the bed (obviously a degrading and humiliating experience), her solution was to fling the tray to make as much noise as possible to get the immediate attention she needed.

Staff follow-up to the incident concluded that the "behavior" presented by E. H. needed to be addressed. The physician obliged by prescribing antipsychotic medications that would have a calming effect to prevent further "acting-out" behaviors.

The family was outraged when they came to visit their mother the following day and she informed them what had transpired. Of course, they objected vehemently to the antipsychotic medication that was prescribed. They insisted their mother never had any "behavioral issues" and her actions were the direct result of the reduced response time of the nursing staff to attend to her immediate biological needs. They threatened to call the appropriate state agencies to report the matter. Needless to say, the prescribed medications were immediately discontinued.

• • •

Since the passage of the NHRA and the OBRA '87, there has not been major legislative reform directed at oversight and enforcement for nursing homes that receive Medicare and Medicaid reimbursement dollars. As has been documented throughout this book, through ample empirical evidence and numerous studies, articles, and government reports from the 1990s to the present, the troubling situation regarding care of elder citizens in skilled nursing facilities continues to exist. With the advent and proliferation of corporate-owned facilities intending maximum profit at all costs, I would venture to say it continues to decline.

Most people are unaware that the 2010 ACA addressed many of these issues. They identify the law with medical insurance, preexisting conditions, and Medicaid dollars. The reality is that the ACA had important language to address the serious situations with skilled nursing facilities. It also incorporated the Elder Justice Act and the Patient Safety and Abuse Prevention Act, which were important for addressing the protection of residents in long-term care facilities from abuse or other crimes. They have been summarized in a brief prepared for the Kaiser Family Foundsation Commission on Medicaid and the Uninsured.[116]

The issues addressed by the ACA are as follows:

* *Ownership information*—Detailed information regarding the individuals or entities that have either direct or indirect ownership of, interest in, or managing control of operations of

---

116 J. Wells and C. Harrington, "Information on Affordable Care Act Provisions to Improve Nursing Home Transparency, Care Quality, and Abuse Prevention," Kaiser Commission on Medicaid and the Uninsured, accessed June 2017, https://kaiserfamilyfoundation.files.wordpress.com/2013/02/8406.pdf.

any nursing home must be disclosed, as well as any other parties that are involved in the governing, managing, administration, operations, finances, or clinical services of that facility.

* *Staffing information*—A national system for collecting and reporting a facility's payroll information must be established by the CMS. In this way the *actual* staffing of direct-care personnel, the number of hours they work, staff turnover, and retention can be tracked for each facility.

* *Facility expenditures*—Cost reports must be redesigned, requiring a breakdown of a facility's expenditures according to specific categories (e.g., direct care, indirect care, capital assets, and administrative services).

* *Nursing Home Compare*—The CMS website which provides consumers with information about facilities, must be revised to add the following information: staffing, health inspections, penalties, and consumer complaints. (See appendix for Nursing Home Compare website information)

* *Complaints*—The CMS must develop a form that standardizes the filing of complaints and the process for resolving them, one that ensures that any complaint filed by a resident and/or his or her representative(s) will not experience retaliation as a result of filing that complaint.

* *Compliance and ethics*—Each facility must establish and operate compliance and ethics programs. These programs would be designed to not only prevent but also detect any violations of a criminal, civil, or administrative nature. A demonstration program to test independent monitoring and oversight of nursing-home chains must be developed by CMS.

The following additional areas of concern were addressed:

- *Penalties*—Civil Monetary Penalty (CMP) requirements must be revised by CMS. These include a means for placing penalties in escrow when nursing homes appeal penalties, and they allow federal penalties to be allocated to programs that would benefit residents.
- *Nursing home closings*—A requirement must be established by CMS for residents to receive a sixty-day written notification informing them of an impending nursing-home closing and providing them with a means of appropriate protection and relocation.
- *Information technology*—A national demonstration project must be established and funded (by CMS) on culture change and the use of information technology to improve resident care.
- *Dementia care and abuse*—Nurse aides must receive training in dementia care and prevention of abuse against nursing-home residents.
- *Background checks*—State programs must be developed and supported by CMS that would conduct national, criminal-background checks on any applicant seeking employment that has direct access to nursing-home residents and/or other recipients of long-term care services.
- *Crime reporting*—Any nursing home or other long-term care facility receiving federal funds (or any employees thereof) must report any suspected crimes against residents to the appropriate law-enforcement agencies.

The CMS has made gains toward implementing the requirements as set forth by the ACA.

These gains are evidenced by the following:

1. The development of new Medicare cost-report forms
2. Improved data collection regarding nursing-home ownership and management and a database that can be readily accessed to search for information on nursing-home owners and managers
3. The development of the Payroll-Based Journal (PBJ) for quantifiable and verifiable staff and census reporting
4. Expanded information regarding complaints and penalties added to the NHC website, with links to nursing-home inspection reports and a searchable database of owners and managers
5. The development of a standardized complaint form
6. Technical assistance provided by CMS to nursing homes on quality assurance and improvement programs

There are major provisions that remain to be implemented, and those include finalizing regulations on full disclosure and transparency of ownership and financial relationships, completing the system for public reporting of nurse staffing information, publicly reporting facility expenditures, and issuing regulations for compliance and ethics programs.

Industry professionals hoped that when all of the requirements as set forth in the ACA were fully implemented, consumers, policymakers, government, and other payer sources would be better able to determine the actual cost of the care provided in these facilities and to assess the quality of the care provided. In the event the ACA is repealed in its entirety, the question left open is if any legislation will address these all-important issues in safeguarding the care of our elder citizens.

In July 2015, the CMS released a 403-page report proposing rule changes aimed at reducing infections and unnecessary hospital readmissions from nursing-home facilities. It also introduced new safety measures and increased quality of care for the approximately 1.5 million recipients of treatment in almost sixteen thousand long-term-care facilities or nursing homes in the country that participate in Medicare and Medicaid reimbursement programs. CMS is the overseeing body, as well as the largest payer source, for long-term-care services in the country. Medicaid accounts for approximately 64 percent of the financial responsibility for nursing-home residents, Medicare approximately 14 percent, and the AHCA—a trade group—for the remaining 22 percent.

As stated by Health and Human Services Secretary Sylvia Mathews Burwell, "When a family makes a decision for a loved one to be placed in a nursing home or long-term-care facility, they need to know that their loved one's health and safety are a priority."[117]

---

117 V. Dickson, "Obama Administration Moves to Strengthen Nursing Home Oversight," *Modern Healthcare*, July 13, 2015, accessed March 2017, http://www.modernhealthcare.com/article/20150713/NEWS/150719975 (hereafter cited as "Obama Administration Moves to Strengthen Nursing Home Oversight").

President Obama addressed the new rules at the White House Conference on Aging on July 13, 2015.[118] Included in the report are these specific changes:

* Training nursing home staff in working with patients who have a diagnosis of dementia and providing specific training in preventing elder-care abuse
* Improving the time line for the care-planning process and involving the IDT in the discharge-plan process, as well as giving consideration to a resident's capacity when considering discharge
* Providing residents with appropriate follow-up information
* Ensuring that all pertinent information and instruction are transmitted appropriately to any facilities or service agencies on the receiving end of the discharge
* Strengthening residents' rights

The response to these changes—which represent approximately $729 million in the first year and $638 million in the second year—was an outcry from AHCA's David Gifford, the senior vice president of quality and regulatory affairs. The response was largely based on the fact that these reforms were not backed with any funding, which places the responsibility on facility owners—the contention being that there is a narrow 1 to 3 percent profit margin that MedPAC calculates for skilled nursing

---

118 "Obama Administration Moves to Strengthen Nursing Home Oversight."

facilities. However, despite what appears to be a narrow margin, SNF owners and corporations have managed to amass millions of dollars in profits from those in their care.

Criticisms included that the proposals fell short of calling for mandatory staffing minimums, which are the root cause for many of the problems in resident care. In addition, critics were seeking more stringent controls for prescribing antipsychotic drugs, which are prevalent in these facilities.

Fast forward to September 2016, when CMS completed the first major overhaul of the 1987 Nursing Home Reform Law, which went into effect in 1991. These changes in regulations, along with the new survey process which examine facility compliance with the new regulations, incorporates portions of legislation from the ACA and the IMPACT Act of 2014, including: Quality Assurance and Performance Improvement (QAPI); Reporting suspicion of a crime; Increased requirements for discharge planning and a section on staff training. They will be phased in concomitant with timetable for the new survey process.

The published ruling is over seven hundred pages, with guidelines and instructions that CMS will set forth over upcoming months and years. The Fall 2016 *LTCCC Journal* discusses both favorable and unfavorable aspects of the new federal ruling.[119]

---

119 R. Mollot, "The Long-Term Care Community Coalition," *The LTCCC Journal* 2, no. 4 (2016), 2–10, www.ltccc.org/news/, (hereafter cited as "The Long-Term Care Community Coalition").

FAVORABLE ASPECTS

RESIDENTS RIGHTS

Residents rights, as previously set forth (see appendix) remain unchanged with some additions in language and clarification. (e.g., the right to be free from abuse, neglect, exploitation, all of which are forms of mistreatment).

CARE PLANNING

Facilities must now develop a baseline plan of care within forty-eight hours of admission, rather than the previously stipulated fourteen days. The baseline plan is meant to include instructions "needed to provide effective and person-centered care that meets professional standards of quality care."[120]This change requires immediate implementation. Another change is that the following essential personnel are added to the care-plan team: a nurse's aide as well as a representative from food and nutrition services.

DISCHARGE PLANNING

When the care team at a facility feels it can no longer meet a resident's needs, it must have sufficient documentation for the reasons, the attempts that were made to meet the needs, and how the receiving facility can meet those needs.

---

120 "The Long-Term Care Community Coalition."

Written notice must be provided to the resident, or designated representatives, explaining the reason for the transfer in language that is clear and easily understood. Notice of impending discharge or transfer must be submitted to a representative of the office of the state long-term-care ombudsman.

If a facility transfers a resident to the hospital and does not anticipate that the resident will return, the facility must follow the above rules and regulations concerning discharge. This is to counteract facilities that intentionally transfer residents they consider to be difficult and for whom they no longer want to care, to the hospital. This practice is commonly known as dumping.

The *LTCCC Journal* reported this statement made by CMS: "We are requiring that facilities develop and implement a discharge-planning process that focuses on the resident's discharge goals and prepares residents to be active partners in post-discharge care, in effective transitions, and in the reduction of factors leading to preventable readmissions." It is also requiring the discharge-planning requirements mandated by the Improving Medicare Post-Acute Care Transformation Act of 2014 (IMPACT Act) by revising, or adding, discharge-planning requirements for long-term care facilities.[121]

CARE FOR TRAUMA VICTIMS
There are provisions that address the needs of trauma victims, such as those who are Holocaust survivors or veterans.

---

121 "The Long-Term Care Community Coalition," 3.

GRIEVANCES

A facility must develop policy for grievances and appoint a grievance officer. Once a complaint is filed, the facility must provide a written response regarding how the issue was investigated, a summary of the results and conclusions, whether or not the grievance was substantiated, and the action or remedy the facility has taken or intends to take to address the issue.

RIGHT TO SUE FOR ABUSE OR SUBSTANDARD CARE

Many facilities previously included clauses in their resident agreements that required residents or their representatives to use arbitration for any dispute they may have had with the facility. This was known as a pre-dispute arbitration clause. Under this system the signee, upon entering the facility, was essentially giving up the right to sue a facility at any time—no matter how egregious the abuse or neglect. The new regulation prevents nursing homes from inserting those clauses, essentially giving residents and their representatives legal recourse to sue a facility in the event of abuse or neglect that results in the resident suffering or dying.

The AHCA, the representative of for-profit facility owners, sued the US government in October 2016 to overturn this ruling. A temporary injunction was issued in November 2016 to stop the ban on pre-dispute arbitration clauses. The organization known as Leading Age, which represents nonprofit providers, did not join in this lawsuit.

An article published in the *New York Times* in August 2017 reported that the Trump administration was advocating dismantling a rule that would have facilitated a nursing-home resident being able to sue a nursing home with greater ease for injuries resulting from substandard care, abuse, or neglect. This would essentially ease the federal regulations that attempted to give residents and their families some recourse in those matters.

The rule the current administration is attempting to dismantle was issued by the Obama administration and prevented nursing homes from having consumers sign an agreement upon admission that any disputes would be resolved through arbitration rather than litigious channels. One could only imagine that, at that delicate and emotional time when nursing-home placement becomes a necessary reality, residents and/or their family members or designated representatives are extremely vulnerable and will sign whatever is necessary in order to facilitate the admission. Furthermore, these clauses are often embedded in the fine print of multipage consumer contracts or admission agreements. One would probably shudder to think their loved one might experience some kind of harm or injury as a result of substandard care, abuse, or neglect in the facility. I would venture to say very few people would consider placement for their loved one if they thought that would become the case. Therefore, the signing of such a consent is not an informed decision.

The reasoning set forth by the Trump administration is that banning arbitration agreements imposes "unnecessary or excessive costs to providers" of nursing-home care. This is another example in which the benefits for ownership supersedes those of the residents.

"Upon reconsideration," the Trump administration said of the proposed nursing-home rule, "we believe that arbitration agreements are in fact advantageous to both providers and beneficiaries, because they allow for the expeditious resolution of claims without the costs and expense of litigation."[122] The money that nursing homes spend on lawsuits could be better used caring for patients, it said. It goes without saying that owners of nursing homes were generally supportive of the proposal. Conversely reaction from others has been extremely against the reversal, resulting in the attorneys general of sixteen states taking stances in strong opposition to the proposal.

UNFAVORABLE ASPECTS

STAFFING

The ruling did not address the serious situation of insufficient staffing in facilities—a major contributor to poor care. No minimum staffing requirements were set forth. The language of the original law stands (that facilities have sufficient staffing to deliver the care and services each resident needs in order to maintain the highest level of physical and psychosocial well-being). The fact that CMS did not pursue a mandate in this area places residents at continued risk for substandard care.

---

122 R. Pear, "Trump Moving to Impede Consumer Lawsuits Against Nursing Homes," *The New York Times*, August 19, 2017, accessed August ,2017, https://www.nytimes.com/2017/08/18/us/politics/trump-impedes-consumer-lawsuits-against-nursing-homes-deregulation.html.

Implementation

The standards and language for classifying problems within a facility remain the same, and no stronger measures were added to enforce the implementation of the changes at the facility level. What is called the F-tag system has been used since the inception of the process as a way for the Department of Health to report on facility deficiencies during its annual survey process. CMS has changed some of the regulatory language, as well as moving categories for different citations, while revising the F-tag system.

The explanation CMS provided was that providers, and even state surveyors, were not properly informed regarding particular categories or infractions, a fact that is hard to understand since these have been in place for twenty-five years. If surveyors were uninformed, how then were they able to conduct their annual surveys and make fair determinations regarding substandard facility conditions? Will they now be better able to identify and cite facilities for infractions and deficiencies that seriously impact the well-being of residents?

Dementia and Antipsychotic Drugging

There has been protective language that has addressed inappropriate antipsychotic drugging—a blatant practice in facilities. Despite these protections over two hundred thousand US nursing-home residents are administered these dangerous drugs for off-label purposes.[123] "Off label" means administer-

---

123 "CMA Comments on Medicare and Medicaid Reforms: Reform of Requirements for Long-Term Care Facilities," Center for Medicare Advocacy, accessed January 2017, www.medicareadvocacy.org/comments-medicare-and-medicaid-programs-reform-of-requirements-for-long-term-care-facilities.

ing a drug for purposes other than it was intended. The new regulation lumps psychotropic medications and antipsychotic medications into one category. The concern is that prescribing pharmaceuticals, especially for dementia patients, will continue, and the care of dementia patients outside of the use of pharmaceuticals will not be addressed. Care for dementia patients outside of drug use may include adjusting the environment so that those capable of walking independently may do so freely without obstructions that may be harmful; adjusting the environment to one that is more soothing; eliminating environmental interruptions that may be discomforting, causing outbursts or other unfavorable behavioral responses (e.g., alarms, flashing lights, overhead pages); matching activities for residents with dementia to the individual's cognitive ability, behavior, and prior interests; providing sufficient activities to alleviate boredom and frustration; ensuring personal needs are met in a timely fashion to avoid discomfort that may lead to outbursts (this is inextricably linked to staffing levels); maintaining consistent staff to promote comfort and familiarity with caregivers; providing more staff supervision; and providing sufficient staff training for staff members assigned to working with individuals with dementia. CMS has announced that they have embarked on a National Partnership to Improve Dementia Care in Nursing Homes. The partnership is amongst federal and state agencies, nursing homes and other providers, advocacy groups, and caregivers for the purpose of finding alternative, non-pharmacological, and a more individualized approach to care for long-term residents with dementia. They report being committed to a 15% reduction in use of antipsychotic medications by the end of 2019. [124] That leaves much room and latitude for their continued use.

Self-Assessment

Facilities are still allowed to monitor and assess themselves in order to identify problems within their facility. Theoretically a facility should be identifying and addressing the issues of concern that impact care, but the reality is that even with oversight many facilities have not been held accountable for identifying or remedying problems—whether the issue is environmental conditions, quality of care, or staffing. What is the incentive for a facility to identify and address issues if there is a monetary cost to rectifying the situation?

Resources for Residents, Families, Ombudsman, and Advocates

Fact Sheet: Medicare Coverage of Skilled-Nursing and Skilled-Therapy Services

Residents receiving therapeutic services (physical therapy, occupational therapy, and speech therapy) are usually discontinued

---

124 "National Partnership to Improve Dementia Care in Nursing Homes Centers on Medicare & Medicaid Services" Last modified 10/25/2017 accessed November 2017, https://www.cms.gov/Medicare/Provider-Enrollment-and-Certification/Survey CertificationGenInfo/National-Partnership-to-Improve_Dementia-Care-In-Nursing-Homes.html

from a service if they no longer demonstrate progress toward their goals or have plateaued, as the facility will not receive reimbursement without continued gains. In fact, there are no specific improvement requirements stipulated to obtain Medicare coverage for skilled-nursing and skilled-therapy services, including physical therapy. Refer to the fact sheet at www.ombuddy.org/medicarecoverageof-skilled-nursing-skilled-therapy-services/ for important information regarding a resident's rights in this area.

There is a move for nursing homes to only provide services for patients in a short-term stay who are receiving rehabilitation services. This is because of the higher reimbursement rate for those receiving rehabilitation. In some instances, patients and their families are being told that after the short-term rehab stay, they will have to go to another facility. However, there are now rulings in place to safeguard against transferring a patient to another facility when the move is unwarranted.

HIGHLIGHTS OF THE INSPECTOR GENERAL'S 2017 WORK PLAN REGARDING NURSING-HOME AND LONG-TERM CARE

This report is based on results of investigations conducted by the office of the inspector general (OIG) of the US Department of Health and Human Services. It identifies serious problems and reports serious deficiencies in the quality of care provided to the residents of nursing homes and long-term-care facilities. The US Department of Health and Human Services is charged with identifying and "protecting the integrity of public health programs and fighting fraud and abuse in Medicare, Medicaid, and other programs."[125]

PIECING TOGETHER QUALITY LONG-TERM CARE: A CONSUMER'S GUIDE TO CHOICES AND ADVOCACY

The November 2016 updated guide provides the most current information, as well as links to outside resources, for residents and families to help them understand how to access the long-term-care services they need and want. The original 2013 national guide was a collaborative effort between the LTCCC and the National Consumer Voice.

The guide can be viewed at: http://ltcombudsman.org/uploads/files/support/piecing-together-quality-long-term-care.pdf

THE NEW SURVEY PROCESS – AN OVERVIEW

Phase One of the new survey process was introduced in November 2016. Many of the changes were more of a clarification or refinement of practices already in place and did not; therefore, require major overhaul of the process. However, there were areas that effected improvement for residents as follows: residents have more decision-making power and input over visitation, who they share a room with, the circumstances surrounding room change, circumstances of discharge, food and dietary preferences and meal times.

---

125 D. De La Mare, "OIG Releases 2017 Work Plan," Long Term Care Leader, accessed January 2017 www.longtermcareleader.com/2016/11/oig-releases-2017-work-plan.html.

The major overhaul of the process occurs in Phase Two when all states will be utilizing the computer-based process for the new LTC survey as of November 28, 2017. The new survey process essentially consists of three parts:

1. The initial pool process
2. Sample selection
3. The investigative process

Phase 2 includes the following focus areas:

* Behavioral Health Services
* Quality Assurance and Performance Improvements (QAPI Plan Only)
* Infection Control and Antibiotic Stewardship
* Physical Environment – smoking policies
* Resident Rights and Facility Responsibilities – Required Contact Information
* Freedom from abuse, neglect, and exploitation – including a requirement for reporting reasonable suspicion of a crime to appropriate enforcement agencies
* Admission, transfer, and discharge rights – Transfer/ Discharge Documentation
* Comprehensive Person-Centered Care Planning – Baseline Care Plan
* Pharmacy Services – Drug regimen review and reporting – review of medical chart, definition of psychotropic medications

* Dental Services – replacing lost dentures
* Administration – Facility Assessment – tied to sufficient and competent staff requirements

The Survey Team Facility Entrance

A brief entrance conference is conducted by the team coordinator with the facility administrator. The team coordinator, and all other surveyors on the team, are supposed to proceed to their assigned units. There is one surveyor assigned the kitchen who conducts a brief visit shortly following the entrance of the team to the facility. A more complete observation of the kitchen will occur at a later stage of the survey.

There are similarities and differences in the new entrance conference. A few revisions include:

* Asking for a list of residents who smoke and their smoking times, which will be used on the first day
* Asking for the number and location of medical storage rooms and carts, which will be used later in the survey
* Asking for updated instructions for the list of residents for the beneficiary notices review.

The "New LTC Survey" process, will require the facility administrator to complete a matrix. The areas of the matrix under consideration are as follows:

❀ Residents Admitted within the Past 30 days

❀ Alzheimer's/Dementia

❀ Mental Illness, Developmental Disability, or Intellectual Disability & No Pre-Admission Screening and Resident Review (also known as PASARR) Level II

❀ Medications – certain medications such as insulin, anticoagulants

❀ Facility Acquired Pressure Ulcers (any stage):

❀ Worsened Pressure Ulcer(s) at any stage

❀ Excessive Weight Loss

❀ Tube Feeding

❀ Dehydration

❀ Physical Restraints

❀ Fall(s)

❀ Indwelling Urinary Catheter

❀ Dialysis

❀ Hospice

❀ End of Life/Comfort Care/Palliative Care

❀ Tracheostomy

❀ Ventilator

❀ Transmission-Based Precautions

❀ Central venous line/Intravenous therapy

❀ Infections

SAMPLE SIZE

The resident sample size for the new survey process will be based on the facility census, with a maximum of 35 residents.

The sampling approach for the new survey process is different from both the Traditional and QIS in that the new survey process includes 70% of MDS pre-selected residents and 30% surveyor-selected residents. Surveyors finalize the sample based on observations, interviews, and a limited record review. The residents selected by the surveyors are expected to include vulnerable residents who are dependent on staff, new admissions within the last 30 days, complaints or facility-reported incidents (FRIs - although to date these are only those that are federally reported)—which would cover any alleged violation involving mistreatment, neglect, abuse, injuries of unknown origin, and misappropriation of property—and any resident who has a significant concern but does not fall into any of the sub-groups just mentioned.

All of the survey processes review facility history information to prepare for the survey. In addition, surveyors will review the offsite selected residents and facility rates during offsite preparation which is similar to the Traditional process.

Unlike the current survey processes, there is no formal tour for the new survey process. Surveyors will begin observing every resident in their assigned area to identify about eight residents for the initial pool process and then will spend about eight hours completing the observations, interviews, and a limited record review for the residents selected for the initial pool process. The surveyors are given autonomy to select residents of their choice for the sample. Part of that review consists of covering a number of quality of life and care areas. During interviews the surveyor is free to determine relevant questions for the interview as long as they maintain the intent of the area. Once the sample is selected, the remainder of the survey is spent conducting investigations for residents, facility tasks and closed records.

UNIT AND MANDATORY FACILITY TASK ASSIGNMENTS

For the new LTC facility survey, tasks are grouped into those required to be investigated on every survey and those only investigated if a concern is identified onsite. Mandatory facility tasks include:

* Dining
* Infection Control
* Skilled Nursing Facility (SNF) Beneficiary Protection Notification Review
* Resident Council Meeting
* Kitchen
* Medication administration and storage
* Sufficient and competent nurse staffing
* Quality Assessment & Assurance/Quality Assurance Performance Improvement (QAA/QAPI)

Soon after the facility entrance, the mandatory facility dining task will require observation of the first scheduled full meal of all dining locations, including trays prepared for residents who remain in their room for the meal. In the event there are more dining areas than surveyors, the dining areas should be prioritized according to the most dependent residents. There should be sufficient dining observations to adequately identify concerns. If it is feasible, the meal for the initial pool of residents who have weight loss should be observed. Subsequent meals should be observed as concerns are identified and after the sample pool is selected.

The new survey process also includes a group interview with residents who are active members of the resident council. The questions asked during the group interview are different from both the Traditional and QIS process.

An important aspect of the new survey process is that the system will select five residents for an "unnecessary medication" review based on information entered by the surveyor during interviews, observations, record review, and information from the MDS.

The selection process considers all psychotropic medications, insulin, anticoagulants, opioids, diuretics and antibiotics, as well as some adverse consequences, including falls, weight loss, and sedation. There are exclusions; for example, a resident would be excluded if they had a diagnosis of Huntington's disease or Schizophrenia and was receiving an antipsychotic. They may also look at new admissions with a broad range of high-risk medications as well as residents receiving a broad range of high-risk medications and adverse consequences

The residents selected for the full medication review will include insulin, an anticoagulant, and an antipsychotic for a resident with a diagnosis of Alzheimer's or dementia, if available.

Another example of an important area for Phase Two implementation is that a facility must have a policy that identifies the circumstances when the facility will assume financial responsibility for loss or damage of a resident's dentures. In this case, the facility may not charge a resident for loss or damage to dentures if indeed the situation has been set forth in the policy as "facility responsibility" It is well known that there are many occurrences of denture loss, for a variety of reasons, in nursing home/skilled nursing facilities. My personal experience with the most egregious of these circumstances has been in a facility that seemed to have an increased number of lost or misplaced dentures as CMI approached. The result was an increase in the number of referrals for dysphagia therapy services to ensure safe and appropriate diet consistencies.

During the survey process, the majority of the surveyor's time should be spent on units observing and interviewing the residents and staff, only using the medical record to corroborate information that is observed and reported. Approximately 40 Critical element (CE) pathways have been developed to assist in guiding the investigation. Surveyors will review to MDS', physician's orders, and care plans initially to guide interviews and observations for the CE pathways. The intention is for surveyors to be completing thorough observations, interviews and limited record review for the residents selected during the initial pool process as they relate to the CE pathways. In the event there is a care areas that does not have a pathway, the interpretative guidance and protocols in Appendix PP will offer the necessary assistance. Interpretative Guidance information is available to assist surveyors in interpreting their observations.

Once the investigation has been completed, surveyors will make a compliance and severity decision for each CE listed for that care area. The CEs are critical components of care—they cover provision of care and services, as well as the facility assessment and care planning.

The Infection Control and Antibiotic Stewardship Program was a continuation of a Phase One requirement as follows: Phase One required that each facility establish and maintain an Infection Prevention and Control Program (IPCP) for the purpose of preventing, identifying, reporting, investigating, and controlling infections and communicable diseases for all residents, staff, volunteers, visitors, and any other individual providing service to the facility under a contractual arrangement. The system will be based on national standards as well as facility assessment. In Phase Two, an "antibiotic stewardship program" was to be implemented as part of the IPCP. The program protocols and a monitoring systems for use of antibiotics.

Among some of the areas slated for implementation in Phase Three are the following:

1. Each facility must designate one, or more than one individual, to serve as an Infection Preventionist (IP) The requirements for that position have been set forth as follows:[126]

    * Have primary professional training in nursing, medical technology, microbiology, epidemiology, or other related field;

---

126 F. Fair "CMS Infection Prevention and Control Updates: Nursing Home F-tags" MS State Department of Health accessed November 2017, http://msphi.org/wp-content/uploads/2017/07/Fair-New-Infection-Control-Requirements-at-F441-6-29-17.pdf

> * Be qualified by education, training, experience or certification;
> * Work at least part-time at the facility; and
> * Have completed specialized training in infection control.
> * Must be a member of the facility's Quality Assessment Committee and will report on a regular basis on the IPCP.
> * While some of these requirements may be new to some facilities, It is expected that many of the requirements for the IPCP policies and procedures may already be part of existing infection control plans.

2. Each facility must develop a compliance an ethics program the entire section of which will be implemented in Phase Three.

3. The Final Regulations includes implementation of QAPI, originally required in the Affordable Care Act. All facilities will be required to develop, implement and maintain an effective and comprehensive, data-driven QAPI program that focuses on systems of care, outcomes of care and quality of life. The facility will be required to maintain documentation and demonstrate evidence of their QAPI program; they will have to maintain a quality assessment and assurance committee that meets at least quarterly. The plan must be presented to the State Survey Agency or Federal Surveyor upon each annual survey period as well as to CMS or upon request during any other survey.

Information on the New LTC survey can be found can be found on the link below – under the heading Downloads: New Long-term Care Survey Process - Slide Deck and Speaker Notes

https://www.cms.gov/Medicare/Provider-Enrollment-and-Certification/GuidanceforLawsAndRegulations/Nursing-Homes.html

In addition, one can go to the National Consumer Voice for Quality Long-Term Care at the links below to view a thorough list of the new regulations as they compare with previous language, side by side comparisons and phases for implementation click on the following under **Rule Resources:**

Part I of the Summary of Key Changes;
Part II of the Summary of Key Changes and,
Side-By-Side Comparison of Revised and Previous Federal Nursing Home Regulations.

To View the full Revision to State Operation Manual (SOM) Appendix PP for Phase 2, F-Tag Revisions, and Related Issues you can click on:
Revised Interpretive Guidelines with a Clickable Table of Contents

http://theconsumervoice.org/issues/issue_details/proposed-revisions-to-the-federal-nursing-home-regulations.

Though we are on the precipice of the anticipated advances that the new regulations and the new survey process will have on the safety, quality of care and lives of our nations long-term care facility residents, it appears that the will and lobbying efforts of providers continue to take precedence. As with other questions in our society today, this should not be a political issue but a moral one. On October 11, 2017, 120 members of the House of Representatives signed on to a letter presented to CMS for the purpose of "reevaluation" of the requirements citing the burden they represent to providers. Of course, there is a possibility that a letter with similar intention can emerge from the Senate. A continued sad fact, indeed. What will it take for this vicious cycle, and denial of decency for our nation's eldest citizens, the vulnerable and dependent among us, to end? When will a higher ground of morality finally prevail? This can be no more evident than the fact that, on this 30th anniversary of **OBRA '87**, CMS is considering backpedaling or delaying implementation of these long overdue revised rules which have been in process for years and the result of numerous articles and studies, some by departments of the government itself. Interested parties (the purveyors of long-term care and their representatives) had ample opportunity to comment or express their concerns prior to CMS' issuing the proposed rule changes.

As previous outlined, CMS stipulated a 3-year timetable to phase in these changes, from 2016-2019. Despite having years of preparation, some have requested that the phase-in-enforcement period be suspended pending a finalized version of a new rule while others call for delaying Phases 2 and 3, the phases with the most critical and crucial changes. In response, CMS has agreed to a moratorium on selected Phase 2 requirements. This is of particular concern as our nation's nursing home residents become older, sicker, increasingly frail, and vulnerable mostly due to dementia and increased physical and other cognitive impairments.

CMS is already considering reneging on the regulations regarding: reporting of abuse and neglect, the QAPI process and discharge notices to long-term care ombudsman. In addition, they have reopened the process for comments on any other areas of the requirements that would result in "reducing the burden" and serve as cost-saving measures to long-term care facilities (i.e., ownership). By doing so they have essentially opened the door to modifying or eliminating many more of the current regulations stipulated in the October 2016 ruling. This process will allow representatives of not-for-profit, but the mainly for-profit facilities, to once again exert their influence and continue their indefatigable efforts to pursue financial gain over quality care for the almost one and a half million nursing home residents. [127]

____

127 Letter summary "Oppose Efforts to Rollback and Delay the Nursing Home Rules" Sign a Letter to CMS! October 31, 2017 The National Consumer Voice for Quality Long-Term Care accessed November 2017, http://theconsumervoice.org/uploads/files/issues/CMS_letter_about_rollback_of_nursing_home_regulations_10-26-17.pdf

CHAPTER 11

Elder Care in America: A Moral Dilemma

• • •

Elder Dignity

At one of the skilled nursing facilities that appeared in other examples in this book, residents with incontinence issues were given a vastly inferior product in order to cut costs (increase earnings). The facility was no longer willing to order pull-ups, similar to the commercial item known as Depends. Instead the facility opted to buy a cheaper, diaper-type product.

Residents were given no advance notice of the change, and only two sizes were ordered: large and extra-large. Those who were smaller in stature, weight, and frame were relegated to wearing diapers that were ill-fitting and uncomfortable. Residents/ patients, families, and staff were appalled. There were dexterity issues involved with opening and closing the adult diapers, and the increased length of time required to open and close the fasteners often resulted in accidents. This was a complete violation of patient dignity and quality of life. Some staff felt so deeply for the residents for whom they cared, they began using personal funds to purchase the pull-up product.

The change in product and resulting dissatisfaction were reported to the administrator and the DON, who merely indicated they knew nothing about the change and did not take any actions. Families were told if they wanted their loved ones to use the pull-up garment, they would have to purchase that product independently. This certainly does not reflect a caring attitude. Yet this company that owns more than forty facilities, and continues to purchase more, is in the business of taking care of people.

Food Quality versus Cost

I met a couple while on vacation in New England with whom I shared similar interests. After getting to know each other, the conversation turned to family. The woman told me her mother had been in a nursing home for a period of time and described the particularly upsetting conditions.

The staff shortages and limited education of the daily caretakers were of concern. However, the issue she found most upsetting was the quality of the food, which she said was so horrible it was almost inedible. Fortunately, a sufficient number of family members and close friends lived near the facility who were able to deliver her mother food on a daily basis. She could not understand how the facility could present such horrible food to people who were either in the process of being rehabilitated or to those sick or frail who lived there on a long-term basis. She had somehow found out that the per-day food allowance for each resident was approximately Three dollars.

Upon further questioning she reported the facility was apparently owned by a major corporate entity that had numerous other facilities under its umbrella, not unlike the facilities in which I work in a different area of the country.

Ignoring Resident's Symptoms and Medication Mismanagement

H. L. is a patient who does not speak any English and has limited family involvement. She had been initially admitted on the short-term rehabilitation unit following a deteriorated condition and mild confusion, with the expectation that she would be returning home. I had seen her in dysphagia therapy and successfully upgraded her diet consistency.

Following the course of her rehabilitation, she was surprisingly moved to the long-term-care unit. I would see her occasionally in the dining room on the floor to which she was transferred when I was treating other residents. After a few weeks, I noticed her condition had drastically changed from someone who was alert, responsive, smiling, and engaging to someone who was oftentimes sleeping through her meals. My colleague and I also noticed that she was coughing intermittently while she ate and drank. I questioned the staff about the resident's obvious change in condition and was told she was not sleeping well at night which resulted in her being sleepy during the day.

I finally approached the unit manager about the issue. She told me she had been in the dining room every day and hadn't noticed any problem. I replied I found that hard to believe; I had been in the dining room every day treating other patients, and H. L. had become sleepier and more lethargic. On this particular day, she seemed to be sweating and was constantly wiping her face and forehead. The nurse merely repeated that there wasn't a problem. I told her I asked the CNA, who reported the woman wasn't sleeping well at night.

The nurse manager went on to question the CNA herself. The CNA reported that the resident was getting up to go to the bathroom many times during the night as the reason she was sleepy during the lunch meal. The nurse manager dismissed the issue in a rather offhand manner, stating that the resident was receiving antibiotics for a urinary tract infection.

However, I persisted. I told her that did not account for the resident coughing or sweating evidenced by her constantly wiping her face and brow. The latter could very possibly be related to reduced tolerance of her present diet consistency, and an evaluation would be warranted. The nurse manager walked away from me, saying nothing further.

On further examination into the situation, it came to light that the resident had been prescribed three sedative-type medications to ensure that she would sleep during the night rather than repeatedly getting up to use the bathroom; a common occurrence with a urinary tract infection. Repeated trips to the bathroom would require the staff to attend to her frequently, as she was not able to independently get to the bathroom.

This was outrageous. It was brought to the attention of the dietitian, the nurse manager, and the director of the rehabilitation department (the latter so that I could obtain an order to evaluate the resident). The following day the dietitian reported to me that at least one of the sedative medications had been discontinued.

● ● ●

OUR ATTITUDE TOWARD, AND TREATMENT of, the elderly, sick, frail, and infirm is just as much a stain on our nation's social conscience as is the history of racial injustice. Major national platforms focus on the care of our children, and the issues of drug addiction, obesity, mental health, and AIDS have been catapulted to a national conversation. However, there is little or no mention of changing our attitude toward elder care and the devaluation of life in advancing years. I postulate that this is an issue of human rights.

An examination of other cultures' treatment and care of the elderly reveals a huge disparity stemming from deeply rooted attitudes and beliefs—not only in philosophy but in use of terminology. Word choices shape our attitudes, and these common phrases connote an attitude of uselessness: "declining years," "over the hill," "old age." A *Wikipedia* definition of "old age" is "nearing or surpassing the life expectancy of human beings and thus the end of the life cycle."[128] I prefer terms such as "elder or older citizens" or "aging parents." These references acknowledge those who have been active, contributing members of our society—far more dignified descriptions.

One need only examine the mores of different cultures to see the effect of deeply rooted philosophical, religious, and ethical beliefs on societal treatment and care of older persons. In China treatment of the elderly encompasses the integral concept of filial piety, or *xiao,* where respect for parents, elders, and ancestors is considered a fundamental virtue.

---

128 *Wikipedia,* s.v. "Old Age," accessed October 2016, https://en.wikipedia.org/wiki/Old_age.

Confucianism outlines the way family members should treat one another and interact, but the philosophy actually goes deeper than that. The Chinese character for filial piety is comprised of a top portion that depicts an old man with a young man underneath, supporting him. The notion of filial piety exists between not just an elder and younger person in the family unit but between any elder and younger person in society as a whole.

This differs significantly from the Western meaning of the words filial piety—the definition of *filial* being *of or due from a son or daughter* and the word *piety* meaning *dutiful and devout.* The Chinese *xiao* can best be described as a relationship based on age or rank, regardless of family ties. Integral to this relationship are attributes of respect, reverence, duty and responsibility, tolerance and patience, provision and welfare, kindness, love and affection, and loyalty.

The English translation of filial piety does not come close to encompassing the virtue that is embodied by the *xiao* character, since *xiao* extends far beyond the individual family unit to society as a whole. The depth to which *xiao* is ingrained in Chinese culture and psyche is best seen by the fact that it extends to one's ancestors and can be described as an ancestral relationship whereby even ancestral worship is valued.

The family does not exist as an independent unit but is a foundation of society. In essence, one's existence and identity are integral to the family and the ancestors from which the family originates; they are interdependent. In the Chinese culture you are nothing without your family and your family name, which is why neglect of one's elders is considered shameful and a blemish on the family name. Furthermore, the *xiao* relationship does not only apply to how one treats elders but to how one addresses them. In essence, filial piety is a moral code of conduct as it relates to family elders and ancestors and is considered fundamental to achieving familial, societal, and social harmony.

In actuality *xiao* did not emanate from the teachings of Confucius alone. Its roots can be found in Taoism and Buddhism, and the influences of Taoism and Buddhism are crucial to understanding the full extent of the tenet. According to Taoist beliefs, *xiao* must flow naturally and be freely expressed—not forced, compelled, or contrived in any way. Compelling *xiao* can result in intense resentment and be entirely counterproductive. In accordance with Buddhist philosophy the virtue of *xiao* is an act of gratitude and repayment of sorts for the parent's boundless, limitless kindness, caring, and love.

The guiding principle of the "Filial Piety Sutra," is that a parent's lifetime of care is considered so difficult to repay that "it can never be compensated even if one were to carry one's parents on the shoulder without putting them down for a hundred or a thousand years."[129] The "Filial Piety Sutra" outlines ten ways

---

129 "Filial Piety Sutra, The Sutra about the Deep Kindness of Parents and the Difficulty of Repaying It" Abstracted from the translation by Upasika Terri Nicholson, as reviewed by Bhikshuni Heng Tao, edited by Bhikshuni Heng Ch'ih and Upasika Susuan Rounds, and certified by Abbot Hua and Bhikshuni Heng Tao. *YBAM Buddhist Digest*, accessed October 2016, http://oaks.nvg.org/filial-piety.html.

in which the mother especially bestows loving-kindness upon the child:

1. Providing protection and care while the child is in the womb
2. Bearing suffering during the birth
3. Forgetting all the pain once the child has been born
4. Eating the bitter herself and saving the sweet for the child
5. Keeping the child dry even if it means she has to stay in the wet
6. Suckling the child at her breast, nourishing, and bringing up the child
7. Ensuring that the child is clean and healthy
8. Always thinking of the child when he or she is away from home
9. Deep care and devotion
10. Ultimate pity (i.e., worry) and sympathy

The tenets of *xiao* and filial piety became mandatory in Confucian fourteenth-century society as a means of achieving social harmony in the war-torn times in which he lived and thus, we identify filial piety with Confucius.

In modern times China is facing challenges to filial piety that are akin to situations in our own country. With the advent of younger people moving from remote areas to the city to find work and working long hours, children are finding it difficult to take time off or use their resources to visit or care for family members. In addition, the Chinese restriction of one child per family has put a tremendous strain on the sole offspring, who must in some cases provide for both parents and grandparents.

Small living spaces in the cities preclude the option of extended family members living under one roof, and older family members who have lived their life in remote areas do not want to move to the city. The result is elderly citizens without means of financial or emotional support and with no way to meet physical needs as they become increasingly frail.

Up to now there has not been a provision for societal elder-care as we know it in China. However, because the concept of filial piety is so ingrained in the Chinese culture and way of life, the government has passed an Elderly Rights Law warning "never to neglect or snub elderly people" and requiring children to visit their parents often, regardless of distance—though there is no definition of "often."[130] In addition adult children are responsible for providing financial, emotional, and physical support for their parents. Parents are even entitled to sue their children if not given adequate financial support.

The government has tried to require businesses to allow time off for children to visit their parents. There are potential penalties for not complying with the law that range from fines to jail. This is a direct contradiction to the basic Taoist principles that *xiao* cannot be forced or compelled, and there are reports of tremendous resentment resulting in neglect and physical and

---

130 M. Meng and K. Hunt, "New Chinese Law: Visit Your Parents," CNN, last modified July 2, 2013, accessed November 2016, www.cnn.com/2013/07/02/world/asia/china-elderly-law/index.html.

emotional abuse. Because of these trends, nursing homes are emerging as acceptable alternatives for elderly care in China.

The influence of the Confucian principle of *xiao* extends to Korea as well, where respect and value for older citizens is considered a fundamental virtue. Reaching sixty years old is considered a rite of passage into old age and is worthy of celebration. Similarly passage into the seventies is marked by significant birthday celebrations. As parents age it is considered honorable, and it is an adult child's duty to care for parents. Placing parents in a retirement home could earn the adult child the label of being an uncaring or bad son or daughter.

The essence of Confucianism followed in Korea can be seen in the following: "Few of those who are filial sons and respectful brothers will show disrespect to superiors, and there has never been a man who is respectful to superiors and yet creates disorder." Confucius wrote this in *Analects*.[131] *The Huffington Post*, in an article on cultures that respect elders, relays the message, "A superior man is devoted to the fundamental. When the root is firmly established, the moral law will grow. Filial piety and brotherly respect are the root of humanity."[132]

It is common practice in the Indian culture to find joint or multigenerational units living together under one roof. The elders become heads of the household, and adult children provide support and cater to the elders' needs. The elders in turn

---

131 W. Chan, *Source Book in Chinese Philosophy* (Princeton, NJ: Princeton University Press, 1963), http://afe.easia.columbia.edu/at/conf_teaching/ct02.html.

132 "Seven Cultures that Celebrate Aging and Respect Their Elders," *The Huffington Post*, last modified May 16, 2015, accessed November 2016, https://www.huffington-post.com/2014/02/25/what-other-cultures-can-teach_n_4834228.html.

play a major role in raising the grandchildren. Elders are placed in high regard: they are sought out for advice on a range of societal, personal, and even financial issues. There is considerable stigma associated with abrogating responsibility by sending elder family members to any type of old-age or living situation outside the home.

The Philippines is like other Asian countries with regard to showing respect to the elder population. This is conveyed both by gestures as well as by the words they use before the person's name. Any younger person addressing an older person is expected to use a specific word (*po* or *opo*) before the name to show respect; to do otherwise is considered to be an act of rudeness.

The word *po* is used to show respect when responding to an older person who has beckoned and is also used in conversation when addressing someone older. The word *ate* is generally used for older sisters or cousins and is said in front of the person's name if she is female. *Kuya* (meaning brother) is used for the male. This term is also used in the workplace to show respect when addressing someone older.

There is also a gesture used to show respect to elders, which is known as "bless" or *mano po*. Upon greeting an elder, the younger person takes the outside of the hand of the elder and places it against his or her own forehead. This action could be considered akin to a priest who places a hand on the forehead as a way of blessing. Therefore, the use of *mano* (the hand) and *po* (bless) is a way for the young to show respect for their elders.

Native American spirituality centers around honor, love, and respect—for the creator, all living things, the earth, and each other. It is the Native American tradition that elders are valued for their knowledge and wisdom and are expected to pass these things down to the younger members of the family. The widely held belief is that elders hold the answers, keep the culture alive, and deserve the utmost respect. This attitude is summed up in a quote by White Feather, a Navajo medicine man: "Native American isn't blood; it is what is in the heart. The love for the land. The respect for it, those who inhabit it; and the respect and acknowledgment of the spirits and the elders. This is what it is to be Indian."[133] There are over five hundred federally recognized Native American tribal communities, each with unique attitudes, traditions, and customs. The prevailing point of view is that elders should be able to remain at home and in their community as they advance in years, known as "aging in place." It is considered to be a continuation of ancient customs of extended and lifelong care for family but also the result of the many year of social isolation and discrimination experienced by Native Americans relegated to living on reservations their entire lives.[134]

An excerpt from the *Inter-Tribal Times*, published in 1994 on the Native American code of ethics says: "Treat every person from the tiniest child to the oldest elder with respect at all times. Special respect should be given to elders, parents, teachers,

---

133 W. Feather, "Native American Beliefs," *Inter-Tribal Times*, last modified October 1994, accessed December 2016, http://www.home.earthlink.net/~tessia/Native.html, (hereafter cited as "Native American Beliefs").

134 C. Printup-Harms, "Aging Elders Among Native American Populations," Niagara County New York, accessed December 2016, http://www.niagaracounty.com/Portals/5/Images/June2010.pdf.

and community leaders. No person should be made to feel 'put down' by you; avoid hurting other hearts as you would avoid a deadly poison."[135]

In most Mediterranean cultures several generations often live under one roof, and there are words to address elders that connote extreme respect and reverence. This is especially true in Greece. In Greek culture the concept of *philotimo* involves generosity, hospitality, and respect for others—especially elders. Furthermore, the culture values seniority: elders are thought to possess wisdom that is an accumulation of years of experience, which is to be respected. This philosophy is epitomized in this quote from BeNeca Ward: "We were taught to respect everyone, especially those who were older and wiser than we were, from whom we could learn."[136]

The Greek word for honor, *hubris,* is associated with renowned Homeric literary works *The Iliad* and *The Odyssey,* dating as far back as the late eighth or seventh century BC and leading to the conclusion that since ancient times honor has been an important consideration in Greek culture. That honor now extends to modern Greek society, where family honor is considered to be a cornerstone that can be destroyed by the action of one family member. However, recent crises in the Greek economy have severely impacted care of its elder citizens. The severe financial measures to maintain functioning society as a whole found pensions for senior citizens slashed by almost 40 percent,

---

135 "Native American Beliefs."
136 B. Ward, "Third Generation Country, A Practical Guide to Raising Children with Great Values," accessed January 2017, https://www.values.com/inspirational-quotes/3002-we-were-taught-to-respect-elders-.

and privately- owned care facilities experienced harsh tax increases, which were passed on as price increases to residents and their families. The programs available for seniors in Greece are mainly adult day care centers and in-home programs, as the country does not have state-funded, long-term-care centers. However, funds for these programs have been affected by significant financial cuts commensurate with the economic crisis, as well as reported mismanagement of funds. There are two organizations that are trying to bridge the gap in this area. The Lifeline Program, which began in 2011, delivers both bags and boxes of food to approximately nine hundred elderly people in Athens on a monthly basis. It also introduced a twenty-four-hour-per-day, seven-day-per-week, pager-alert system whereby an elderly person at home can contact someone in the event of an emergency. It also operates a national helpline for those elderly citizens who are neglected or abused or who are experiencing medical or family issues. A program established in 2005, known as 50+, promotes elder citizen rights and provides incentives for them to be active in society.

There may be further challenges to come for the elder citizens in Greece if the financial climate results in deeper pension cuts, shrinking social-program funding that may all but disappear.[137] The situation in present-day Greek society is a disheartening and stark contrast to the philosophy of ancient Greece, where it was considered a sacred duty of the children to look

---

137 D. Lelvada, "How Two Organizations Are Bringing Hope and Care to Greece's Elderly," *The Huffington Post*, last modified January 10, 2017, accessed May 2017, www.huffingtonpost.com/entry/greece-elderly_us_561d6ed5e4b0c5a1ce60f1d2.

after the elderly. When societal finances are strapped, support for the citizens that contributed to that society are scrapped.

There has been an interesting development in France regarding care of elders that is unrelated to an underlying filial-piety-type philosophy. In 2004 an Elderly Rights Law passed, due largely to statistical information reporting that the highest rate of suicide was among "pensioners" (sixty-two deaths per week). Adding impetus to the legislation was a horrific situation in which fifteen thousand elderly people died as a result of a crippling heat wave. Their bodies, in a staggering number of cases, were unclaimed for weeks because their families were on annual holiday.

Article 207 of the French Civil Code requires children to honor and respect their parents, pay them an allowance, and provide or fund a home for them; repercussions for not doing so can result in fines or imprisonment. The law stipulates that it is a crime if children do not keep abreast of their parents' medical conditions if they live alone and that they must intervene if parents become ill. According to a parliamentary report, "it is not acceptable that children exonerate themselves from all responsibility for their aged parents."[138]

As in the United States, in France there is a fascination—and almost idolization—of youth. Dr. Renee Arnaud-Castigliioni, head of the psychiatric service for the elderly at Marseilles hospital, says that society "overvalues the image of youth at the

---

138 K. Wilsher, "French Forced to Care for Elderly Parents," Fairfax Digital, last modified February 16, 2004, accessed October 2016, http://www.theage.com.au/articles/2004/02/15/1076779835689.html, (hereafter cited as "French Forced to Care for Elderly Parents").

expense of the elderly."[139] In the United States, the youth culture is highly valued along with independence, individualism, and self-reliance. This, along with the Protestant work ethic (i.e., if you're no longer working, your societal value is significantly diminished), impacts attitudes toward our older citizens. What younger people fail to realize when they are looking askance at an elder person, is that they are looking, hopefully, and their future selves: a concept that is understandably hard to grasp. Who among us ever thought we would actually reach this age?

From a technological viewpoint, the older generation has also lost its usefulness. Contemporary literacy and access affords us the ability to use search engines to find information. What young people miss in procuring information in this way is the flavor and the context of rich family stories and traditions that other cultures value as the wisdom associated with knowledge. The information gleaned from a search engine cannot give advice. It creates a false conception that information and personal knowledge result in better decisions than the wisdom that comes with years of experience, which only an older person can provide. As Jared Diamond so beautifully states, "The repositories of knowledge are the memories of the old people."[140]

To American youth and many young adults, older people are an intrusion, a nuisance, an annoyance, and a burden. In our fast-paced, immediate-gratification society, where we have no time for ourselves—let alone others—there is no place for the time, effort, and patience needed to care for our aging citizens.

---

139 "French Forced to Care for Elderly Parents."
140 "French Forced to Care for Elderly Parents."

While there may be more TV commercials depicting care, medication, and consideration for parents with Alzheimer's, dementia, or other ailments associated with older citizens, they are still few and far between. It is so much easier to find a place for senior adults to stay and to assume they will be cared for in a respectful, decent, and dignified manner.

The problem is not a US issue alone. While it is not integral to our culture—as it is with some others—to respect or value older people, taking care of an aging population is statistically becoming a worldwide problem. The elderly population in Japan is growing exponentially. Statistics report that by the year 2020, 7.2 percent of the Japanese population will be eighty years old or older. Supplies necessary for older citizens are selling in greater numbers than those for babies, and pension funds are expected to dwindle or dry up entirely.

In 2000 there were six hundred million people in the world aged sixty and over. This number is expected to increase to 1.2 billion by 2025 and 2 billion by 2050. Today about two-thirds of all older people are living in the developing world, and by 2025 it is predicted to be 75 percent. In the developing world, the eighty-plus population, considered as the very old, is the fastest growing population.

In China awareness of an ever-increasing older population resulted in an unprecedented 2015 government ruling to increase the family allowance of children from one to two. As it is around the world, where advances in medicine are increasing life expectancy, the result is an increase in the aging population for which nursing homes are emerging as an option for elderly care. This is compounded by a trend in China, as around the world (e.g., Japan and India), where young people want privacy and a home of their own.

Jeremy Hunt, the secretary of the National Health Service (NHS) in Great Britain, gave a speech entitled "Elderly Treatment 'National Shame.'" He said that England should be ashamed of how it treats the elderly and that, according to the Campaign to End Loneliness, eight hundred thousand chronically lonely elderly people existed in English society. Family members who do not visit the elderly leave them feeling isolated, and people should examine how they treat their own parents and grandparents.[141]

He said, "If we are to tackle the challenge of an aging society, we must learn from this and restore and reinvigorate the social contract between generations."[142] Hunt has also stated that health care has to be more human and patient centered and not system and bureaucracy centered. This holds true for our country as well. It is counterintuitive that the nursing-home industry has become a business, rather than a patient-care model.

Being "elderly" is a generalized term that creates stereotypical thinking not applicable to everyone who falls in an age range. There are people who are alert, vital, and active in the later stages of life—some who continue to work until their seventies

---

141 O. Wright, "'Our National Shame': Health Secretary Jeremy Hunt Blasts British Society's Neglect of Its Elderly," *Independent*, last modified October 17, 2013, accessed October 2016, http://www.independent.co.uk/news/uk/politics/our-national-shame-health-secretary-jeremy-hunt-blasts-british-society-s-neglect-of-its-elderly-8887532.html.

142 D. Blackburn, "Jeremy Hunt Calls for 'Profound Transformation in the Culture' of the NHS," *The Spectator*, November 19, 2013, accessed January 2017, https://blogs.spectator.co.uk/.

and eighties. Appropriate intervention is more than a function of chronological age. It includes issues of mental health and capacity, physical health, and social isolation.

The General Assembly of the United Nations established what it termed as an Open-Ended Working Group (OEWG) on Ageing[143] in December 2010 for the purpose of protecting the human rights of older persons. It is hoped that the results will be undertaken as part of the world human rights convention.

In the meantime, we should do better in this country. As the conversation on national health care addresses the much-needed health care for our citizens, there also needs to be a national conversation about meeting the needs of our elder citizens in a more dignified and respectful manner. This conversation must be without consideration for the accumulation of astronomical profits by a few who, along with the rest of us, will become sick, old, and infirm one day and will want better for themselves and their families.

---

143 [131]"Open-Ended Working Group on Ageing," United Nations Human Rights Office of the High Commissioner, accessed April 2017, https://social.un.org/ ageing-working-group/.

EPILOGUE

...

Speech Therapy: From Then to Now

When I initially began working as an SLP in skilled nursing facilities, it took tremendous effort to convince administrators and directors of rehabilitation departments that if the results of an evaluation indicated a patient or resident required speech, language, or dysphagia therapy, a schedule of treatment once or twice a week did not constitute sufficient services.

At the same time, physical and occupational therapy, which were reimbursable expenditures, were being offered on a daily basis. When called to a facility, I would always present the analogy that if an individual visited a doctor and required a prescription for medication, the medication would be dispensed based on the patient's condition and need, not based on what the patient was willing or able to pay.

I developed a strategy of placing the person on program for a minimum of twice per week and after several weeks would have to convince administration that three times would be more beneficial for effecting improvement. The additional time was usually approved, but it was often an uphill battle.

That all changed in the early 2000s, when completion of an MDS included therapy minutes as a calculation for reimbursement and speech therapy minutes were included in that calculation. At that time I worked for a facility that had been purchased by a major player in the corporate world of nursing-home ownership. The corporate regional director of rehabilitation, a rather gregarious and affable physical therapist with whom I enjoyed a comfortable working relationship, repeatedly joked with me that people might actually start to care about speech therapy as much as I did and that I was now free to pick up anyone I wanted for the program. It was no longer a fight to convince the powers that be that people needed speech/language/dysphagia therapy services; now I had to give evidence of why some people were not candidates for services.

On occasion at that facility, I would actually receive lists of names of patients from the director of the rehabilitation department questioning why I had not picked up particular patients for programs. This was overcorrection to an extreme level, as some of the patients on those lists were long-standing, ventilator-dependent patients who presented with limited responsiveness and were clearly not capable of participating in a therapy program.

Moving forward to the present, with RUGS categories for Medicare and the prescribed periods of CMI throughout the year for calculating Medicaid reimbursement rates, the situation has only exacerbated exponentially. On the favorable side, there is no longer a fight to provide speech/language/dysphagia therapy services, and individuals are getting therapy when they might not otherwise have received it at all. However, the pendulum has swung too far in the opposite direction. It is now not necessarily about providing service to those in need but providing service to anyone possible for purposes of financial gain.

It wouldn't be fair to conclude without giving credit to the many professionals and staff workers at every level within these facilities, from facility administrators all the way down the chain to therapists and support staff, who care deeply for the patients or residents and who, despite the difficult conditions and many financial pressures, truly try to provide the best care and advice possible, based on their expertise and knowledge. I speak for myself—but I know this is true of many of my colleagues—in saying that it is difficult not to become both professionally and personally disheartened. I struggle with the idea of providing speech, language, and dysphagia rehabilitation therapy, as well as improving the quality of life for long-term-care residents amid the insatiable profit motive that seems to become more challenging to navigate with each passing day.

It is also important to mention that family members and loved ones also want the best for the individual placed within the facility. As a result, they seem at times jaded by the negative information and many "horror" stories they hear, are distrusting and disbelieving of that advice, or have expectations beyond what may seem reasonable, based on the patient or resident's condition or status.

I have seen those who not only refuse to take the advice offered, arguing every step of the way, but engage in actions that are in exact opposition to the advice, thereby causing or having the potential to cause negative impact or consequences. Included here are a few examples.

● ● ●

Feeding

A.R. was a patient at a facility where I was working. When she was admitted she was in an advanced state of dementia and had recently had a feeding tube inserted due to her poor swallowing ability that was characterized by holding food in her mouth, limited intake, and aspiration pneumonia. I was told she had been in that facility many times previously and that as her dementia worsened feeding had become increasingly difficult with each subsequent admission.

I went to evaluate the resident and found her with poor responsiveness and inability to open her mouth when I attempted to feed her. Since she had only recently been given the feeding tube, I tried repeatedly. When I met with her husband, he suggested that she would do better in his presence as well as in the hours approaching lunchtime when she would be out of bed. I agreed and began seeing the patient as he suggested.

Within a two-week period, A. R. began to improve in her response, and I began feeding her small amounts. After a little over a month, we began feeding her small amounts of a lunch meal, which she was able to consume with encouragement, coaxing, strategies, and much assistance from her husband, who visited most of each and every day.

After several months had passed it appeared the plan for her to return home was becoming more remote. As she was no longer a candidate for the short-term-rehabilitation unit, she was moved to another unit that focused on long-term-care residents.

Mr. R continued to be a constant companion and daily visitor, taking more of the responsibility for feeding his wife. However, she began to decline, and feeding her seemed to be less and less successful. The nurses on the unit would discourage Mr. R. from feeding when his wife appeared less awake and less able to accept and safely tolerate the food. As a result, Mr. R would become adamant, rude, and somewhat verbally abusive to the staff. He became increasingly dissatisfied with the facility and ultimately transferred her elsewhere.

Several months later, I began working at another facility through a different agency contract. Lo and behold I came across Mr. R and his wife, A. R. He told me that since he had been at this new facility, staff members were not feeding his wife anything by mouth, and he was not happy. I was surprised he had not become adamant in his insistence as he had at the previous facility. I had spoken with the speech therapist who evaluated A. R. on admission, and she said the resident was not responsive; therefore, she did not recommend any attempts for feeding. Because I had previous experience with both Mr. R and A. R., I convinced nursing and the director of the rehabilitation department that I should try again.

Mr. R could be a charming man, well dressed, and fastidious. He expressed being highly appreciative of the fact that I was making the effort to try and have his wife begin to eat food by mouth.

I began as I had before, with Mr. R in attendance assisting and encouraging his wife to open her mouth and swallow. After about a week and a half, it appeared it was becoming an increasingly unsafe situation. A. R. became increasingly lethargic, drifting into sleepy states while feeding and holding the food in her mouth for longer and longer periods of time. Eventually some of it would ooze out of her mouth. On other occasions, we could get her to take a small sip of liquid, which would help her swallow the food in her mouth. Sessions lasting thirty to forty-five minutes were successful in having her accept no more than up to half of a teaspoon three times, and there was continuing concern about food left in her mouth, which, when she was in a resting state, could ooze down her throat resulting in choking.

I educated Mr. R that it had become unsafe to continue attempting to feed her, that she was receiving sufficient nutrition via the tube, and advised against him giving her anything by mouth. However, he was observed by nursing staff on two occasions attempting to give his wife a liquid nutritional drink, and I observed it on an additional occasion.

As a result, the team called a meeting with Mr. R. The director of nursing, the social worker, the nurse on the unit, and I provided education about the risks and consequences of continuing to offer anything by mouth and advised Mr. R against doing so.

His response was similar to the response he had in the previous facility when similarly advised. He became adamant, rude, and verbally aggressive toward me and everyone on the team. The meeting ended with Mr. R indicating he was looking for an alternative placement for his wife. He ultimately moved his wife to another facility in the area.

Struggle of a Professional Who Became a Caregiver

I worked with a dietitian at a facility in which there was a unit with patients who were ventilator dependent. We both spent a considerable amount of time on that unit and discussed our encounters with family members who were insistent on having their loved ones eat when it was clearly medically contraindicated.

After a few years of working together, the dietitian's husband became very ill and was hospitalized. When I visited him in the hospital she told me medical professionals had him on very severe dietary restrictions. I was shocked when she told me that, despite the medical advice, she was giving him small amounts of a bagel with cream cheese and chocolate. I couldn't believe my ears.

This came from someone fully knowledgeable about the risks and consequences of providing food that was contraindicated. She told me she couldn't help herself; he wanted it and begged her to give it to him.

I reminded her of all the families with whom we worked, how difficult it was when we provided education about food restrictions, and the frustration we felt *when they did not take the advice, sometimes providing food that could cause harm. She said she knew, but she loved him and he was begging her.*

Family Insistence

I had an experience while working at another facility during this same time period that also had a unit devoted to patient's dependent upon ventilators. There was a female patient in her eighties who was not very responsive and was receiving G-tube feeding. It was recommended I evaluate her for her potential to eat.

Upon completing the evaluation, I determined that it would be too risky to place any food inside the patient's mouth. She was extremely weak and presented with limited responsiveness. I had the opportunity to meet with the patient's son, who introduced himself as a doctor, and advised him of my findings.

During my next visit to the facility, I was called to the conference room, where I was met by both the administrator and assistant administrator. The administrator, a rather loud, boisterous, bullying type of man, asked me about my evaluation findings for the patient. After I told him the results, he proceeded to point his finger at me and yell, "You will evaluate the patient for food." I told him I would not, because it was not safe. He insisted again and continued to yell at me, saying that the patient's son would call the state if I didn't. My final answer was that if I put food in the woman's mouth and she aspirated—with the potential for very dire consequences—the patient's son would be suing me, and the administrator would merely say, "I don't know. She's the professional clinician. She evaluated the patient." I left the facility that day and arranged to work full-time at the other facility where I was working. I tendered my resignation on my next visit to that facility.

● ● ●

FINAL THOUGHTS

As of the writing of this book, the continual changing landscape of health care in the United States creates confusion and anxiety among those who are in the position of seeking care options for their loved ones, those responsible for loved ones residing in care facilities, or individuals who are living in care facilities. Though there is little talk in our society about the aging process, its associated conditions, and the cost of death and dying, it is incumbent upon us as individuals, and society in general, to begin the conversation—especially in light of the increase in our aging population.

The issue of investor-owned, for-profit, health-care corporations was reported on by the Institute of Medicine based on a 1986 study entitled "The Changing Structure of the Nursing Home Industry and the Impact of Ownership on Quality, Cost, and Access."[144] The article not only examined the for-profit paradigm for hospitals but delved into issues that relate to nursing homes that have been occurring since the 1970s. The results were astounding. The article reported that the nursing facilities under for-profit corporations, as well as those that were part of a chain of ownership, spent fewer dollars on direct patient care, resulting in reduced quality of care. Results of additional studies through the years were consistent with that study.

---

144 C. Hawes and C. D. Phillips, "The Changing Structure of the Nursing Home Industry and the Impact of Ownership on Quality, Cost, and Access," last modified 1986, accessed May 2017, https://www.ncbi.nlm.nih.gov/books/NBK217907/.

For the first time, an analysis was undertaken in 2011 of the ten largest for-profit nursing-home chains for the years between 2003 and 2008. It compared for-profit ownership with not-for-profit. The findings were consistent with previous reports. Researchers found that for-profit facilities had the following:

1. The lowest staffing levels
2. The highest number of deficiencies identified by public regulatory agencies
3. The highest number of deficiencies causing harm or jeopardy to residents

The GAO issued a report in 2010 that reported on what is known as special-focus facilities. These are the ones that have been identified by the CMS as the poorest-performing facilities across the country. Its findings included these:

1. These facilities are more likely to be part of a chain and for-profit compared to other facilities.
2. They have fewer registered nurses per resident per day.
3. They are ranked lower on the CMS five-star rating system.[145]

---

145 "Poorly Performing Nursing Homes: Special Focus Facilities are Often Improving, but CMS's Program Could Be Strengthened," US Government Accountability Office, last modified April 19, 2010, accessed May 2017, http://www.gao.gov/products/GAO-10-197.

The GAO issued another report in 2011 that focused on facilities that were purchased by the top-ten private-equity firms between 2004 and 2007 and found the following:

1. They had more total deficiencies than not-for-profit facilities.
2. They reported lower total nurse-staffing ratios.
3. They showed capital-related cost increases and higher profit margins compared to other facilities.[146]

One can easily conclude that in general the type of ownership of a particular facility has implications for the quality of care being delivered to its patients and residents.

As previously stated, the ACA, in recognizing the seriousness of the issue, included a provision for full disclosure and transparency of the details of nursing-home facility ownership to the CMS and for that information to be available to the public. In this way families would have a better chance of making more informed choices about where to place their loved ones and have some knowledge and expectancy about the care that would be delivered. Considering the seriousness of the situation with nursing-home ownership and its impact on quality of care, any future legislation should address this all-important issue.

The question remains: despite the knowledge and information regarding for-profit ownership and the impact on care, why

---

146 "Nursing Homes Private Investment Homes Sometimes Differ from Others in Deficiencies, Staffing, and Financial Performance," US Government Accountability Office, last modified July 2011, accessed May 2017, http://www.gao.gov/new.items/d11571.pdfancial.

has this type of ownership been allowed to skyrocket? In the past few years in my area alone, almost every facility in which I have worked that was not-for-profit, or those that I know of that were privately owned, has been bought out by a handful of these corporations. I know of one company that, because it may no longer be able to purchase facilities in New York State, has reached out across the country, recently buying a dozen facilities in a South-Central State and major investor in that company has ownership in facilities in three other states in another area of the country.

What does this mean? The proliferation of these companies across the country has serious implications for the ever-growing issue of the care of our nation's elder citizens. It is incumbent upon our nation's policy makers to devise reimbursement systems that mandate that the dollars are spent on providing a level of care that is commensurate with decency and respect for our elders and removes the loopholes that allow owners huge profit margins.

The way we care for this population reveals much about our society and our underlying values about the quality of life that each individual deserves as he or she continues life's journey. The funding, staff development and training, research, and continued oversight of our long-term-care facilities will determine the future of this population—of which most of us will become a part. It is imperative that the issue of nursing homes and rehabilitation centers becomes part of the national conversation on health care.

During the final editing stages of this book, the *New York Times* dated September 24, 2017, had a feature article entitled "A

Preventable Descent into Suffocating Chaos" [147] that reported on a tragedy in a Florida nursing home during Hurricane Irma that resulted in multiple deaths (14) of our elder citizens. As were many others, I was as horrified by the news in real time as I was again when reading the *Times* article. What was most tragic to me was that, after the headline and subsequent article, it became just another passing news story with little lingering interest or news attention. I deliberated on how or whether I should include the information in this book as just another example of how we disregard the lives of residents in nursing homes.

Finally, I came across the response from the LTCCC, whose reports I referenced throughout this book. After pondering the issue, I decided that it couldn't be said more appropriately than it was by Richard Mollot, the executive director of the coalition.

"We are extremely distressed by reports of multiple resident deaths at the Rehabilitation Center at Hollywood Hills nursing home. Nursing homes are charged with safeguarding vulnerable residents twenty-four hours a day, seven days a week. Each facility that is licensed by Medicare and/or Medicaid makes a promise to residents and their loved ones that it will provide sufficient staffing, care, and other services necessary to ensure that every resident is safe, comfortable, and able to live with dignity. In addition to the promises made to individuals, these promises extend to the American public, which pays for a substantial portion of nursing-home care, including care provided by this for-profit nursing home. Safeguarding residents during hurricanes and other

---

147   E. Gabler, S. Fink, and V. Yee, "A Preventable Descent into Suffocating Chaos" *The New York Times*, September 24, 2017.

natural disasters is a longstanding integral component of nursing-home requirements in this country. We believe that it should go without saying that a nursing home has the available resources, and its staff sufficient knowledge, to take the steps necessary to avoid residents being placed in dangerous or precarious situations. However, because, too often, facilities do not provide sufficient staff or services that meet minimum standards, the federal government has established specific requirements and guidelines for ensuring that residents are protected under emergency circumstances." [148]

The State of Florida began the process to suspend the license of the Hollywood Hills nursing home and close an assisted living facility operated by the same owner of the Hollywood Hills nursing facility back in December of 2016. A notice was filed to deny Floridian Gardens, that assisted living facility, renewal of its license based on deficiencies related to staffing, training, administration of medication, inattentiveness, food service, and even an instance of sexual assault.

In January 2017, the action to deny the license renewal was challenged and remains pending. The loss of the lives of the eleven residents who suffocated in the sweltering heat in the aftermath of the hurricane has been added to the state's charge against the facility owners. Sadly, the owners were successful in winning a slight reprieve prior to the hurricane, and on August 24, 2017 the ban against Floridian Gardens admitting new patients was lifted.

---

148 "Statement on Post-Irma Nursing Home Deaths," The Long-Term Care Community Coalition, accessed October 2017, http://nursinghome411.org/statement-hurricane-irma/.

Following Hurricane Irma local police authorities, together with other agencies, initiated a criminal investigation into the deaths of eight of the residents whose body temperatures were measured in excess of 108 degrees Fahrenheit.

The lawyers retained by the ownership of the facilities continue to further challenge the state's move to close Hollywood Hills nursing home and has called the action "illegal and improper." [149]

A final ruling was published (Federal Register Vol. 81, No. 180) on September 8, 2016. It specified a regulation effective November. 16, 2016, to be implemented by November 15, 2017, regarding Emergency Preparedness requirements for all providers and suppliers that participate in receiving Medicare and Medicaid reimbursement. For further information on the emergency preparedness regulations issued by CMS, please visit https://www.cms.gov/Medicare/Provider/Enrollment-and-Certification/SurveyCertEmergPrep/Emergency-Prep_Rule.html).

The full Emergency Preparedness regulations was issued on June 2, 2017 as Appendix Z of the State Operations Manual which contains the guidelines and survey procedures for the Emergency Preparedness Final Rule.[150]

---

149 R. Mills, "Florida Moves to Close Second Facility Run by Owner of Nursing Home Where Eleven Died," *USA Today*, September 28, 2017, https://www.usatoday.com/story/news/nation-now/2017/09/28/florida-moves-close-second-facility-run-owner-nursing-home-where-11-died/715239001/.

150 Appendix Z, Emergency Preparedness Final Rule Interpretive Guidelines and Survey Procedures Centers for Medicare & Medicaid Services June 2, 2017 accessed November 2017, https://www.cms.gov/Medicare/Provider-Enrollment-and-Certification/SurveyCertificationGenInfo/Downloads/Survey-and-Cert-Letter-17-29.pdf.

APPENDIX

· · ·

Skilled Nursing Facility versus Nursing Home

The fundamental difference between a skilled-nursing facility and a nursing facility is the certifying or regulatory body that oversees the reimbursement. The terms are often used interchangeably; colloquially speaking when people refer to a nursing home, they generally mean a skilled-nursing facility. However, even the Medicare website uses the terms interchangeably.

This is readily noted on the Nursing Home Compare website, which helps individuals search and compare facilities. (website information included in appendix list of websites) Though the title of the website contains the words "nursing home," it actually compares skilled nursing facilities. Skilled nursing facilities are certified by Medicare for a prescribed period of time, up to one hundred days, as well as by Medicaid, by ensuring they meet specific guidelines. Furthermore, the department of health in each state is responsible for holding these facilities responsible to meet the criteria set forth by regulatory agencies.

Criteria for Establishing a Skilled Nursing Facility

* The facility must have a hospital-transfer agreement in place in the event a resident or patient is in need of emergency services or restorative or rehabilitative care.
* Skilled-nursing and rehabilitation staff evaluate, observe, manage, and provide treatment. One example of skilled-nursing care might be IV injections. An example of rehabilitative care would be physical, occupational, or speech

therapy. Care that can be given by nonprofessional staff (e.g., CNAs) does not fall within the realm of a skilled service.

* When Medicare certifies a facility as a skilled-nursing facility, it is saying it ensures the facility has the staff and equipment to provide needed skilled-nursing care, rehabilitation services, and other related health services.

Skilled-nursing and rehabilitation staff includes the following:

* A medical director to provide oversight for clinical quality and medical policies and/or practices
* Registered and licensed practical nurses
* Licensed physical and occupational therapists
* Speech-language pathologists
* Audiologists

WHAT ARE NURSING HOMES?

A nursing-home environment is one that provides what is commonly referred to as custodial care (i.e., ADLs, which include getting in and out of bed, assistance with meals and/or feeding, bathing, dressing, and using the bathroom). This care is administered by trained paraprofessionals (e.g., CNAs). Certified professional health-care workers, nurses, and doctors may be available or on staff, but the individual resident is not generally in need of that level of expertise.

In addition nursing homes that are freestanding facilities are not regulated by the federal government and, therefore, are not under the same strict Medicare and Medicaid guidelines as skilled nursing facilities. Nursing homes are associated with, and often run by, charitable organizations (e.g., the church or various orders of nuns, like the Carmelite Sisters).

Skilled-nursing services are offered in both hospital-based facilities and in freestanding facilities. A skilled-nursing facility can either be affiliated with a hospital or it can be a stand-alone building (freestanding). Freestanding buildings are usually part of a nursing home that covers skilled-nursing facility services reimbursed by Medicare. This type of facility also covers the care provided to long-term residents who are either private pay, subsidized by Medicaid, or in possession of their own long-term-care insurance. For the most part, only a small portion of Medicare recipients are part of the total resident population in a freestanding nursing home.

Nursing Homes or Nursing Facilities

Medicare also covers nursing-home care for certain people who require custodial care, meet a state's means-tested income and asset tests, and need the level of care offered in a nursing home.

* Nursing-home residents have physical or cognitive (short- or long-term) impairment and require twenty-four-hour care during their stay.

* The cost of staying in a nursing home can be several thousand dollars per month. Without any other choices, people have been known to exhaust their financial resources due to the high cost of nursing-home care. Medicaid will cover long-term stays in nursing home for eligible individuals for life. However, Medicaid requires that the individual does not retain assets beyond a certain level. Therefore the individual is required to either "spend down" his or her assets to the required level or to protect those assets through an attorney who specializes in elder law. There is a look-back period that Medicaid uses to determine whether the individual intentionally has protected assets, including the transferal of assets to another party. The look-back period can range from five to seven years.

* The primary caregiver in a certified nursing home is a CNA, who has limited formal training. Therefore, most of the resident care in nursing facilities is not provided by skilled, licensed personnel. The nature of the work for the majority of these direct caregivers is task oriented, meaning they are assigned specific tasks to perform for numerous residents on a specific unit.[151]

---

151 "The Difference between Nursing Homes and Skilled Nursing Facilities," As You Age, January 2017, http://www.asyouage.com/Difference_Between_Nursing_Homes_And_Skilled_Nursing_Facilities.html.

*P*ERTINENT *Q*UESTIONS FOR *C*ONSIDERATION
The following questions are intended for those who might already have a loved one in a skilled-nursing facility or rehabilitation center or who are considering placement in a facility for themselves or a loved one. Individuals should not be reluctant to ask questions. After all this is an environment in which they or their loved one will be staying, whether briefly or long term. The information contained in the previous chapters should illustrate why asking these questions is important.

1. What are some of the demographics of the patient population as it relates to age, average length of stay (if considering long-term), cognitive status, or psychological impairment? In other words is there a preponderance of patients with Alzheimer's or dementia versus more psychological-type impairments?

2. Is the loved one being given therapy for what is necessary or appropriate for him or her, or does the motive seem to be the facility's income? Is more therapy given during a specific time of the year that might correspond to increasing reimbursement statistics?

3. Is the loved one's frequency and duration of therapy being determined by his or her condition, the facility's needs, or by insurance?

4. Is the timing of the loved one's discharge from the facility based on what is actually best for him or her or on what may increase the facility's bottom line?

5. Who is available to provide psychosocial support services, if needed, and what is that person's schedule of availability?
6. Who is attending to the loved one's medical needs—a medical doctor, a nurse practitioner, or a physician's assistant? Who is signing off on care? How often will the loved one be seen?
7. What are the facility's staffing policy and ratios for days, evenings, and weekends? How many RNs are on duty at any particular time? How many CNAs are on the unit where the loved one would be staying?
8. How does the facility handle behavioral issues and patient/resident disagreements?
9. What insurance does the facility accept?
10. How does the facility engage patients/residents in activities? What activities are available, and for what portion of the day are patients sitting idly without any form of activity?
11. What were the facility's survey results? Were there any deficiencies? Was the facility found to have any deficiencies that were related to patient care or quality of life? If yes, what steps has the facility taken to address those issues?

Resident Bill of Rights
More detailed information regarding resident's rights within the SNF or NF.

The Right to Be Fully Informed
There shall be full disclosure regarding the following information:

* Available services and the charges for each service
* Facility rules and regulations, including a written copy of resident rights
* Address and telephone number of the State Ombudsman and state survey agency
* Access to State survey reports and the facility plan of correction
* Advance notification of room or roommate changes
* Assistance in the event of sensory impairment (vision, hearing)
* The right to receive information in a language they understand (any language that is their predominant language which includes Braille or Sign Language)

RIGHT TO COMPLAIN

The resident is free to:

* Present grievances to staff or any other person, without fear of reprisal for which the facility will promptly make efforts to resolve those grievances;
* Complain to the ombudsman program
* File a complaint with the state survey and certification agency

RIGHT TO PARTICIPATE IN ONE'S OWN CARE

This includes the right to:

* Receive adequate and appropriate care without discrimination
* Be informed of all changes in medical condition
* Participate in their own assessment, care-planning, treatment, and discharge
* Refuse medication and treatment
* Refuse chemical and physical restraints
* Review one's medical record
* Be free from charge for services covered by Medicaid or Medicare

RIGHT TO PRIVACY AND CONFIDENTIALITY

This is afforded to residents under any circumstance but is necessary as follows:

* Private and unrestricted communication with any person of their choice
* During treatment and care of one's personal needs
* Regarding medical, personal, or financial affairs

RIGHTS REGARDING TRANSFERS AND DISCHARGES

The resident has the right to remain in the nursing facility unless a transfer or discharge:

* is necessary to meet the resident's welfare;
* Is appropriate because the individual's status has improved and she or he no longer requires nursing home care;
* Is needed to protect the health and safety of other residents or staff;
* Is required because the resident has failed, after being appropriately notified, to pay a facility charge for an item or service that was provided at their own request
* If discharge is required, the resident shall receive thirty-day notice of transfer or discharge which includes the reason, effective date, location to which the resident is being transferred or discharged. The resident also has the right to appeal the impending discharge and may

contact the state long-term care ombudsman. The facility shall provide the resident with the ombudsman's contact information
* All preparations to ensure that the transfer or discharge is safe shall be completed by the facility

RIGHT TO DIGNITY, RESPECT, AND FREEDOM

The expectation in this area is as follows:

* To be treated with consideration, respect, and dignity
* To be free from mental and physical abuse, corporal punishment, involuntary seclusion, and physical and chemical restraints
* Freedom for choosing activities, schedules and health care decisions as per your personal interest
* To feel safe and secure for your person, property, possessions and money

RIGHT TO VISITS

Shall include persons of a resident's choice as well as:

* The individual's personal physician
* Representatives from the state survey agency and ombudsman programs
* Relatives, friends

* Representatives or organizations or individuals who provide health, social, legal, or other counseling services
* Ultimately, the residents has the right to refuse visitors

RIGHT TO MAKE INDEPENDENT CHOICES

To the best of the individual's ability, the resident is free to:

* Make personal decisions on a daily basis such as clothing choices and how to spend free time
* Reasonably and appropriately accommodation one's needs and preferences
* Select the physician of their choosing
* Participate in community activities, both inside and outside the nursing home
* Organize and participate in a Resident Council
* Manage one's own financial affairs

SIX NEW STAR RATINGS

1. Percentage of short-stay residents/patients admitted to a skilled-nursing facility who stayed less than or equal to one hundred days and who had an emergency-room visit as an outpatient (based on Medicare claims)
2. Percentage of short-stay residents who were successfully discharged to the community and who were not readmitted to a hospital or another skilled-nursing facility within thirty days—some facilities are extending this to sixty days—of discharge or who did not die (based on Medicare claims)
3. Percentage of short-stay residents who were rehospitalized following admission to the skilled-nursing facility, including observation stays (based on Medicare claims)
4. Percentage of short-stay residents who made improvement in physical function and locomotion (per MDS)
5. Percentage of long-stay residents—stays of greater than or equal to 101 days—whose ability to move independently worsened (per MDS)
6. Percentage of long-stay residents who received an anti-anxiety or hypnotic medication (as per MDS)

States Accepting Expanded Medicaid Coverage

1. Alaska
2. Arizona
3. Arkansas
4. California
5. Colorado
6. Connecticut
7. Delaware
8. Hawaii
9. Illinois
10. Indiana
11. Iowa
12. Kentucky
13. Louisiana
14. Maryland
15. Massachusetts
16. Michigan
17. Minnesota
18. Montana
19. Nevada
20. New Hampshire
21. New Jersey
22. New Mexico
23. New York
24. North Dakota
25. Ohio
26. Oregon

27. Pennsylvania
28. Rhode Island
29. Vermont
30. Washington
31. West Virginia

Information/Websites

By using search engines, individuals can find organizations, websites, and newspaper articles reporting on individual nursing homes and nursing-home corporations, as well as their owners. In addition, many of these websites, as well as other articles, describe a variety of nursing-home experiences for patients who are either currently in, or have been in, nursing homes.

It is important to be aware of potential harm, so one can recognize it at the earliest moment and accordingly advocate, whether personally or on behalf of a loved one. There are additional helpful websites included in Chapter 4 of this book.

Of special note is a site, Families for Better Care, that reports on nursing homes that have been added to a federal watch list for the most egregious infractions and worst quality of care. The site's list is updated monthly.

- www.AsYouAge.com
- FATE (Foundation Aiding the Elderly)—www.4fate.org
- Families for Better Care – familiesforbettercare.com
- LTCCC (Long Term Care Community Coalition) – ltccc. org/ or nursinghome411.org/
- ProPublica Nursing Home Inspect – http://projects.propublica.org/nursing-homes
- www.assisted-living411.org
- www.nextstepincare.org
- www.nursinghome411.org
- Billian's Health Data Portal – www.definitivehc.com/ Billians (Billian's Health Data Portal has been acquired

and integrated into Definitive Health Care, thus the URL incorporates both names)

* National Consumer Voice – theconsumervoice.org
* Leading Age – leadingage.org
* Administration on Aging (AOA) – agingcare.com
* American Health Care Association (AHCA) – Https:www.ahcancal.org
* Careconversations.org
* Long-term Care – senior.com
* Health Finder – healthfinder.gov
* Nursing Home Compare – http://www.medicare.gov/nursinghomecompare/search.html?
* Office of Long-Term-Care Ombudsman Programs – www.ltcombudsman.org

ABBREVIATIONS AND ACRONYMS

Terminology in any area with which one is unfamiliar can be confusing. Health care, long-term care in particular, has its own jargon and share of abbreviations. This list is not meant to be an exhaustive list of all the terminology one will encounter, either as a reader or in a real-life setting. However, it is meant to help readers as a reference for this book as well as to familiarize them with unfamiliar terms. When working with a facility, always feel free to ask the meaning of an abbreviation or acronym. The *Annals of Long Term Care: Clinical Care and Aging and the 2014 CMS Statistics* report from the US Department of Health and Human Services was used as a guide in completing this list.

ADE or ADR—Adverse Drug Event or Adverse Drug Reaction
As the name implies, an ADE or ADR is an unwanted event or reaction that could cause harm from a particular medication.

ADLs—Activities of Daily Living
This refers to the many self-care activities that are performed each day (e.g., bathing, dressing and undressing, toileting, getting into and out of bed, walking—also called ambulating—and eating). In the long-term-care setting, the degree of help an individual requires to perform any of these activities is rated from maximum to no assistance (independent).

ARD—Assessment Reference Date
This is the MDS date by which evaluations and assessments must be completed and scored on the document.

CAA—Care Assessment Area
The CAA refers to the framework that is used to review the areas of concern that are triggered by the MDS. This is a more in-depth analysis of the concern areas.

CAT—Care Area Trigger
These are the conditions that are based on the MDS and that are usually found to require further evaluation before an intervention on the care plan is completed.

CCP—Comprehensive Care Plan
This instrument is used to state a patient's/resident's problems and goals and to set forth the interventions to address and remediate those problems within the facility. It is essentially a contract of the plan of care.

CDC—Centers for Disease Control and Prevention
This federal agency provides the guidelines for the treatment and prevention of infectious diseases.

CMI—Case-Mix Index
A classification system where the care offered to individual residents is classified into categories based on the intensity of the

care and services provided. It considers diagnoses, conditions, treatments, and assistance with Activities of Daily Living (ADLs).

CMS—Centers for Medicare & Medicaid Services
This is the federal agency within the US Department of Health and Human Services that administers and oversees Medicare programs and works in concert with state governments that administer and oversee Medicaid programs.

CPR—Cardiopulmonary Resuscitation
This is a process that is used in an attempt to revive an individual in the event the person stops breathing or the heart stops beating.

CVA—Cerebrovascular Accident
This is a term used when an individual has a stroke.

DOA—Date of Admission

DOB—Date of Birth

DOH—Department of Health

DM—Diabetes Mellitus

EMR—Electronic Medical Record

ESRD—End-Stage Renal Disease
This is a disease affecting kidney function.

G-Tube—Gastric Feeding Tube
This is a device used to provide nutrition to patients who cannot otherwise successfully or safely receive food by mouth or who require alternative methods of feeding to supplement their oral intake. The process of being fed by a G-tube is called enteral feeding, or tube feeding. Tube feeding can be administered over a period of time or in individual administrations, known as bolus feeding.

H&P—History and Physical
The history and physical is customarily completed on an individual's admission to a facility.

HIPAA—Health Insurance Portability and Accountability Act
This 1996 federal law was passed to ensure and protect an individual's medical information from anyone other than those given the authority to have knowledge of the patient's condition.

IDDM—Insulin-Dependent Diabetes Mellitus

IDT—Interdisciplinary Team

IV Therapy—Intravenous Therapy
An IV allows needed liquid to be introduced to the body directly through a vein and is considered to be the fastest way to infuse the body with liquids or medication.

LPN or LVN—Licensed Practical Nurse or Licensed Vocational Nurse

LTC—Long-Term Care
A facility designed to accept residents who are intended to stay for an undetermined period of time.

MDS—Minimum Data Set (current version 3.0)
This is the federally mandated instrument that is completed to assess all residents in a Medicare- and Medicaid-certified, approved facility. The instrument is designed to identify and record an individual's problem areas and the treatment provided to address those areas, which are then reported for reimbursement purposes.

MI—Myocardial Infarction
This is another term for a heart attack.

NF—Nursing Facility

NG Tube—Nasogastric Intubation
In this circumstance, the tube is passed through the nose, past the throat, and into the stomach for the purpose of providing nutrition. It is intended as a temporary measure with a limited time frame.

NKA—No Known Allergies

NP—Nurse Practitioner

OBRA—Omnibus Budget Reconciliation Act

This is more commonly referred to as the Nursing Home Reform Act of 1987, the purpose of which was to establish federal standards for the delivery and quality of care to nursing-home residents.

OT—Occupational Therapy or Occupational Therapist
(Note: A COTA or OTA is a Certified Occupational Therapy Assistant or Occupational Therapy Assistant.)

PA—Physician's Assistant

PDP—Prescription Drug Plan

PICC Line—Percutaneous Intravenous Central Catheter
This is alternatively referred to as a peripherally inserted central catheter, which is used when introduction of fluids or medication needs to be intravenously provided over a prolonged period of time.

PPS—Prospective Payment System
This is the system of payment adopted to pay nursing-home facilities.

PT—Physical Therapy or Physical Therapist
(Note: A PTA is a Physical Therapy Assistant.)

QI—Quality Indicators
These are areas identified within the facility that are particularly concerning in their impact on patient care. The purpose is to

develop strategies and interventions to prevent negative results for patients.

QCI—Quality of Care Indicators
These are resident centered and are derived from calculations from downloaded MDS data, as well as data collected on-site during the state survey process (e.g., things like the number of residents who developed in-house pressure ulcers).

RAI—Resident Assessment Instrument
This is a standardized measure that is used in determining a complete picture of a resident's strengths and weaknesses. It has three components: the MDS 3.0, the CAA process, and the RAI Utilization Guidelines, which is a guide explaining how to use and apply the RAI.

RN—Registered Nurse

RUG—Resource Utilization Group
These are the groups into which nursing-home Medicare patients are categorized based on the services and therapy minutes they require as needed by their medical condition and functional status. This is the basis for determining the nursing-home reimbursement rate.

SLP—Speech and Language Pathologist

SMI—Supplementary Medical Insurance

SNF—Skilled Nursing Facility
This includes any nursing-home facility certified to accept Medicare and Medicaid reimbursement.

SQC—Substandard Quality of Care

SSA—Social Security Administration

ST—Speech Therapy or Speech Therapist

TJC—The Joint Commission
Formerly known as the Joint Commission on the Accreditation of Healthcare Organizations (JCAHO), the commission evaluates the level of health care hospitals and nursing homes provide and certifies that the institutions meet and adhere to specific standards of care.

TPN—Total Parenteral Nutrition
This occurs when an individual's nutritional needs are met intravenously, and he or she does not receive nutrition by any other means. It may also be referred to as peripheral parenteral nutrition (PPN) when the nutrition is delivered through a vein in a limb rather than through a central vein.

WNL or WFL—Within Normal Limits or Within Functional Limits
This is used to describe test results, an examination, or a function that is within the range that is expected. Age and gender are taken into consideration.

Abbreviations Used for Administering Medication

QD—Once a day

QShift—Once per shift

BID—Twice a day

TID—Three times a day

QID—Four times a day

QHS—At bedtime

PRN—Per resident need or when needed (e.g., pain medication)

AC—Before meal

73 Federal Register 25918, at 25923, May 7, 2008, accessed August 2017, http://frwebgate2.access.gpo.gov/cgi-bin/PDFgate.cgi?WAISdocID=FAFj8E/0/2/0&WAISaction=retrieve.

73 Federal Register 46416, at 46422, August 8, 2008, accessed August 2017, http://frwebgate1.access.gpo.gov/cgi-bin/PDFgate.cgi?WAISdocID=HcQhNJ/0/2/0&WAISaction=retrieve.

2008 Agency Financial Report, Section III-23 Health and Human Services, 11/17/2008; Updated 12/08/2008 accessed March 2017, https://www.hhs.gov/about/agencies/asfr/finance/financial-policy-library/agency-financial-reports/index.html See Archive of HHS Financial and Performance Reports

"2014 CMS Statistics," US Department of Health and Human Services, accessed September 2017, https://www.cms.gov/Research-Statistics-Data-and-Systems/Statistics-Trends-and-Reports/CMS-Statistics-Reference-Booklet/Downloads/CMS_Stats_2014_final.pdf.

Abramo, A., and Lehman, J. "How N.Y.'s Biggest For-Profit Nursing Home Group Flourishes Despite a Record of Patient Harm," ProPublica, last modified October 27, 2015, accessed October 2016, https://www.propublica.org/article/new-york-for-profit-nursing-home-group-flourishes-despite-patient-harm.

"Accountability in Nursing Home Abuse and Neglect," Finkelstein and Partners, accessed November 2016, http://www.lawampm.com/blog/nursing-home-abuse-and-neglect/2016/03/18/accountability-in-nursing-home-abuse-and-neglect.

Amon, M. "How a Long Island Nursing Home Empire Got Its Way," *Newsday*, January 5, 2008.

"Analysis of Bundled Payment," RAND Corporation, accessed February 2017, https://www.rand.org/pubs/technical_reports/TR562z20/analysis-of-bundled-payment.html.

Appendix Z, Emergency Preparedness Final Rule Interpretive Guidelines and Survey Procedures Centers for Medicare & Medicaid Services June 2, 2017 accessed November 2017, https://www.cms.gov/Medicare/Provider-Enrollment-and-Certification/SurveyCertificationGenInfo/Downloads/Survey-and-Cert-Letter-17-29.pdf.

"Appropriateness of Minimum Nurse Staffing Ratios in Nursing Homes," Executive Summary Report to Congress Phase II Final, Vol I December 2001 Abt Associates, Inc. accessed June 2017 http://theconsumervoice.org/uploads/files/issues/CMS-Staffing-Study-Phase-II.pdf.

"A Profile of Older Americas: 2013," Administration for Community Living, accessed September 2017, https://www.acl.gov/sites/default/files/Aging%20and%20Disability%20in%20America/2013_Profile.pdf.

Atchley, R. C. *Social Forces and Aging* (Belmont, CA: Wadsworth Publishing, 1994)

Baggot, D. "The Bundled Payment Title Wave: Recap and Insight from the Fourth National Bundled Payment Summit," Oregon Healthcare News, July 7, 2014, accessed August 2017, http://www.revolvy.com/main/index.php?s=Bundled%20payment&item_type=topic.

Baucus, M. "Call to Action," American Health Lawyers Association, accessed February 2017, https://www.healthlawyers.org/Members/PracticeGroups/TaskForces/HRE/Documents/CalltoAction_HealthcareReform.pdf.

"Bill Promotes RNs in Long-Term Care," *The American Nurse*, June 14, 2017, http://www.theamerican nurse.org/2014/11/04/bill-promotes-rns-in-long-term-care/.

Blackburn, D. "Jeremy Hunt Calls for 'Profound Transformation in the Culture' of the NHS," *The Spectator*, November 19, 2013, accessed January 2017, https://blogs.spectator.co.uk/.

Boccuti, C., Casillas G., and Neuman, T. "Reading the Stars: Nursing Home Quality Star Ratings, Nationally and by State," The Henry J. Kaiser Family Foundation, accessed March 2017, https://www.kff.org/medicare/issue-brief/reading-the-stars-nursing-home-quality-star-ratings-nationally-and-by-state/.

Bowblis, J. R., and Brunt. C.S. "Medicare Skilled Nursing Facility Reimbursement and Upcoding," *Health Economics*, accessed February 2017, http://citeseerx.ist.psu.edu/viewdoc/download?doi=10.1.1.403.6500&rep=rep1&type=pdf.

Breyer, M. "New Chinese Law Will Let Elderly Parents Sue Children for Neglect," *Mother Nature Network*, March 19, 2013, accessed September 2016, http://www.mnn.com/earth-matters/politics/stories/new-chinese-law-will-let-elderly-parents-sue-children-for-neglect.

Butler, R. N. *Why Survive: Being Old in America* (New York: Harper and Row, 1975)

"Care Area Assessment (CAA) Process and Care Planning—RAI Manual 3.0 Chapter 4," Centers for Medicare & Medicaid Services, accessed January 2017, https://www.ahcancal.org/facility_operations/Documents/UpdatedFilesRAI3.0/MDS%203.0%20Chapter%204%20V1.03%20August%202010.pdf.

Casale, A. S., Paulus, R.A., Selna, M.J., Doll M.C., Bothe Jr., A.E., McKinley, S., Berry, A., Davis, D.E., Gilfillan, R.J., Hamory, B.H., and Steele Jr., G.D., "ProvenCare[SM]: A Provider-Driven Pay-for-Performance Program for Acute Episodic Cardiac Surgical Care," *Annals of Surgery* 246, no. 4 (2007): 613–21, discussion 621–23, accessed February 2017, https://www.ncbi.nlm.nih.gov/pubmed/17893498.

"Case Mix Prospective Payment System for SNFs Balanced Budget Act of 1997,"

CMS.gov accessed October 2017, https://www.cms.gov/Medicare/Medicare-Fee-for-Service-Payment/SNFPPS/index.html

Chan, W. *Source Book in Chinese Philosophy* (Princeton, NJ: Princeton University Press, 1963), http://afe.easia.columbia.edu/at/conf_teaching/ct02.html.

"Chapter 4: A Path to Bundled Payment around a Hospitalization," Medicare Payment Advisory Commission, June 2008 accessed February 2017, 67.59.137.244/chapters/Jun08_Ch04.pdf.

"China's Elder Care Law—A Struggle for One-Child Families," *VOA Press Asia,* July 18, 2013, accessed October 2016, https://www.voanews.com/a/china-elder-care-law-a-struggle-for-one-child-families/1704200.html.

"Choosing A Medigap Policy: A Guide to Health Insurance for People with Medicare," Centers for Medicare & Medicaid Services and National Association of Insurance Commissioners, accessed March 2017, https://www.medicare.gov/Pubs/pdf/02110-Medicare-Medigap.guide.pdf.

Cimiotti, J. P., Aiken, L.H., Sloane, D.M., and Wu, E.S. "Nurse Staffing, Burnout, and Health-Care Associated Infection," *American Journal of Infection Control* 40, no. 6 (2012): 486–90. Accessed September 2017, doi:10.1016/j.ajic.2012.02.029.

"CMA Comments on Medicare and Medicaid Reforms: Reform of Requirements for Long-Term Care Facilities," Center for Medicare Advocacy, accessed January 2017, www.medicareadvocacy.org/comments-medicare-and-medicaid-programs-reform-of-requirements-for-long-term-care-facilities.

"CMS Proposes Changes to the Comprehensive Care for Joint Replacement Model, Cancellation of the Mandatory Episode Payment Models and Cardiac Rehabilitation Incentive Payment Model," Centers for Medicare & Medicaid Services, accessed November 2016, https://www.cms.gov/Newsroom/MediaReleaseDatabase/Fact-sheets/2017-Fact-Sheet-items/2017-08-15.html.

Coll MD, P. "Medical Terms and Abbreviations Commonly Used in Long-Term Care," *Annals of Long Term Care: Clinical Care and Aging* March 2011; 19(3): 20–24, accessed April 2017, https://www.managedhealthcareconnect.com/.../ medical-terms-and-abbreviations-com.

"Comparison of Benefits of Different Types of MLTC Plans," Independent Consumer Advocacy Network, accessed October 2017, http://icannys.org/icanlibrary/comparison-of-benefits-in-different-types-of-mltc-plans/.

"Confucian Teaching: Three Confucian Values: Filial Piety (Xiao)" Asian Topics: Excerpt from: Chan, "A Source Book in Chinese Philosophy Chan" Wing-tsit ed., (Princeton, NJ: Princeton University Press, 1963), Analects 12, accessed Feb 2017 http:// afe.easia.columbia.edu/at/conf_teaching/ct02.html

Connole, P. "Nursing Facilities Embrace Short-Stay Residents," *Provider Magazine*, July 2010, accessed March 2017, http:// www.providermagazine.com/archives/archives-2010/ Pages/0710/Nursing-Facilities-Embrace-Short-Stay-Residents.aspx.

Connolly, C. "For This Health System, Less Is More. Program That Guarantees Doing Things Right the First Time, for Flat Fee, Pays Off," *Washington Post*, March 31, 2009. HighBeam Research accessed September 2017, https://www.highbeam. com/publications/the-washington-post-p5554/mar-31-2009

Corbin-Jallow, S., and Moore, R. "CBO Memorandum: Projections of Expenditures for Long-Term Care Services for the Elderly," Congressional Budget Office, http://www.dtic.mil/get-tr-doc/pdf?AD=ADA399651.

Cromwell, J., Dayhoff, D. A., and Thoumaian, A. H. "Cost Savings and Physician Responses to Global Bundled Payments for Medicare Heart Bypass Surgery," *Health Care Financing Review* 19, no. 1 (1997): 41–57, accessed February 2017, https://www.ncbi.nlm.nih.gov/pubmed/10180001.

Cromwell, J., Dayhoff, D.A., McCall, N.T., Subramanian, S., Freitas, R.C., Hart, R.J., Caswell, C., and Stason, W. "Medicare Participating Heart Bypass Demonstration," Centers for Medicare & Medicaid Services, accessed April 2017, https://www.cms.gov/Research-Statistics-Data-and-Systems/Statistics-Trends-and-Reports/Reports/downloads/oregon2_1998_3.pdf.

Cutter, M. "Under Pressure," *The ASHA Leader,* accessed April 2017, leader.pubs.asha.org/issue.aspx?issueid=930256.

De La Mare, D. "OIG Releases 2017 Work Plan," Long Term Care Leader, accessed January 2017 www.longtermcareleader.com/2016/11/oig-releases-2017-work-plan.html.

Dickson, V. "Obama Administration Moves to Strengthen Nursing Home Oversight," *Modern Healthcare,* July 13, 2015 accessed March 2017, http://www.modernhealthcare.com/article/20150713/NEWS/150719975

DiNapoli, T. P. "Nursing Home Surveillance," Office of the New York State Comptroller, accessed October 2016, https://www.osc.state.ny.us/audits/allaudits/093016/15s26.pdf.

Duhigg, C. "At Many Nursing Homes, More Profit and Less Nursing," *New York Times*, September 23, 2007, accessed September 2017, http://www.nytimes.com/2007/09/23/business/23nursing.html?pagewanted=all&_r=0.

Edmonds, C., and Hallman, G.L. "Cardiovascular Care Providers: A Pioneer in Bundled Services, Shared Risk, and Single Payment," *Texas Heart Institute Journal* 22, no. 1 (1995): 72–76. Accessed May 2017, https://www.ncbi.nlm.nih.gov/pmc/articles/PMC325213/

Ellsworth. B. "The Beginning of the End of RUGs As We Know It" Health Dimensions Group April 28, 2017 accessed November 2017, http://healthdimensionsgroup.com/beginning-end-rugs-know/

Encyclopedia of Aging Online, s.v. "Nursing Homes: History," The Gale Group, Inc. 2012 accessed August 2016, http://www.encyclopedia.com/education/encyclopedias-almanacs-transcripts-and-maps/nursing-homes-history.

Epstein, A. *The Challenge of the Aged* (New York: Alfred A. Knopf, 1929)

"Extendicare Health Services Inc. Agrees to Pay $38 Million to Settle False Claims Act Allegations Relating to the Provision of Substandard Nursing Care and Medically Unnecessary Rehabilitation Therapy," US Department of Justice, accessed September 2017, https://www.justice.gov/opa/pr/extendicare-health-services-inc-agrees-pay-38-million-settle-false-claims-act-allegations.

"Facts about the Sentinel Event Policy," Joint Commission, last modified February 13, 2017, https://en.wikipedia.org/wiki/Sentinel_event.

Fair, F. "CMS Infection Prevention and Control Updates: Nursing Home F-tags" MS State Department of Health accessed November 2017, http://msphi.org/wp-content/uploads/2017/07/Fair-New-Infection-Control-Requirements-at-F441-6-29-17.pdf

FastStats-Nursing Home Care CDC/National Center for Health Statistics U.S. Department of Health & Human Services Last updated May 3, 2017 accessed October 2017, https://www.cdc.gov/nchs/fastats/nursing-home-care.htm

"Filial Piety Sutra, The Sutra about the Deep Kindness of Parents and the Difficulty of

Repaying It" Abstracted from the translation by Upasika Terri Nicholson, as reviewed by Bhikshuni Heng Tao, edited by Bhikshuni Heng Ch'ih and Upasika Susuan Rounds, and certified by Abbot Hua and Bhikshuni Heng Tao.

YBAM Buddhist Digest, accessed October 2016, http://oaks.nvg.org/filial-piety.html.

Fitzwater, A. "The Pros and Cons of Switching to a Medicare Advantage Plan," eHealth, accessed January 2017, https://medicare.com/medicare-advantage/the-pros-and-cons-of-switching-to-medicar-advantage/.

"Five-Star Quality Rating System Technical Users' Guide," Centers for Medicare & Medicaid Services, Updated August 2016, accessed November 2016, https://www.cms.gov/Medicare/Provider-Enrollment-and-Certification/CertificationandComplianc/downloads/usersguide.pdf.

"From the House of Delegates: Help in Responding to 'Productivity' Issues on Its Way," *PT in Motion,* July 9, 2014, accessed February 2017, http://www.apta.org/PTinMotion/NewsNow/2014/7/9/HoDProductivity/.

Gabler, E., S. Fink, and Yee, V. "A Preventable Descent into Suffocating Chaos" *The New York Times,* September 24, 2017.

Goroll, A. H., Berenson, R.A., Schoenbaum, S.C., and Gardner, L. B. "Fundamental Reform of Payment for Adult Primary Care: Comprehensive Payment for Comprehensive Care," *Journal of General Internal Medicine* 22, no. 3 (2007): 410–15. Accessed March 2017, https://www.ncbi.nlm.nih.gov/pmc/articles/PMC1824766/

Gosfield, A. G. "Making PROMETHEUS Payment Rates Real: Ya' Gotta Start Somewhere," Robert Wood Johnson Foundation, last modified June 2008, accessed June 2017, www.rwjf.org/en/library/research/2009/06/what-is-prometheus-payment-.html.

Greenwood, E. "Controversial 'Filial Piety' Law Comes into Effect in China," *Global Post*, July 2, 2013, accessed February 2017 https://www.pri.org/stories/2013-07-02/controversial-filial-piety-law-comes-effect-china.

Gregory, S. "The Nursing Home Workforce: Certified Nursing Assistants," AARP Public Policy Institute, accessed March 2017, http://www.aarp.org/home-garden/livable-communities/info-2001/aresearch-import-688-FS86.html.

Haber, C., and Gratton, B. *Old Age and the Search for Security: An American Social History* (Bloomington: Indiana University Press, 1994)

Harrington, C., and Millman, M. "Survey of State Staffing Standards Included in a Report Prepared for the Henry J. Kaiser Family Foundation," University of California, San Francisco, accessed April 2017, https://books.google.com/books?isbn=0763707538.

Hawes, C., and Phillips, C. D. "The Changing Structure of the Nursing Home Industry and the Impact of Ownership on Quality, Cost, and Access," last modified 1986, accessed May 2017, https://www.ncbi.nlm.nih.gov/books/NBK217907/.

"Health Facilities Consumer Information Systems Long-Term Care Facility FAQs," California Department of Public Health, accessed May 2017, https://cdph.ca.gov/.

Hernandez-Medina, E., Eton, S., and Hurd, D. "Training Programs for Certified Nursing Assistants," AARP Public Policy Institute, accessed July 2017, https://assets.aarp.org/rgcenter/il/2006_08_cna.pdf.

"High-Risk Series: An Update," US Government Accountability Office, accessed September 2017, https://www.gao.gov/assets/240/237065.pdf.

"History of the 19th Century American Poorhouses," The Poorhouse Story, accessed August 2017, http://www.poorhousestory.com/history.htm.

Hussey, P. S., Eibner, C., Ridgely, M.S., and McGlynn, E.A. "Controlling US Health Care Spending—Separating Promising from Unpromising Approaches," *New England Journal of Medicine* 361, no. 22 (2009): 2109–11, accessed June 2017, https://www.ncbi.nlm.nih.gov/pubmed/19907037.

"Improving Medicare Post-Acute Care Transformation Act"- IMPACT Act of 2014 H.R. 4994 113th Congress (2013-2014) accessed October 2017, Congress.gov https://www.congress.gov/bill/113th-congress/house-bill/4994

"Institutional Special Needs Plans (I-SNPs)," Centers for Medicare & Medicaid Services, accessed May 2017, https://www.cms.gov/Medicare/Health-Plans/SpecialNeedsPlans/InstitutionalSNP.html.

Johnson, L. L., and Becker, R. L. "An Alternative Health-Care Reimbursement System—Application of Arthroscopy and Financial Warranty: Results of a Two-year Pilot Study," *Arthroscopy* 10, no. 4 (1994): 462–70, discussion 471–72, accessed May 2017, http://bostonshoulderinstitute.com/wp-content/uploads/2015/03/Johnson-et-al-1987-An-Alternative-Healthcare-Reimbursement-System-Arthroscopy-and-Financial-Warranty.pdf.

Kander, M. "How Medicare Reimbursement Works in Skilled Nursing Facilities," *The ASHA Leader* 19 (2014): 26–27, leader.pubs.asha.org/article.aspx?articleid=1878428.

Klauber, M., and Wright, B. "The 1987 Nursing Home Reform Act," AARP, accessed September 2016, http://www.aarp.org/home-garden/livable-communities/info   2001/the_1987_nursing_home_reform_act.html.

Knickman, J. R., and Snell, E.K. "The 2030 Problem: Caring for Aging Baby Boomers," Health Services Research, accessed September 2017, https://www.ncbi.nlm.nih.gov/pmc/articles/PMC1464018/#b13.

Krantz, M. "Wall Street Banks Ace Fed's Severe Stress Test" *USA Today Money Section B* June 24, 2016

Lee, T. H. "Pay for Performance, Version 2.0?" *New England Journal of Medicine* 357, no. 6 (2007): 531–33, accessed May 2017, www.nejm.org/doi/full/10.1056/NEJMp078124.

Lee, H. Y., Blegen, M.A., and Harrington, C. "The Effects of RN Staffing Hours on Nursing Home Quality: A Two-Stage Model," *International Journal of Nursing Studies* 51, no. 3 (2014): 409–17.

Lelvada, D. "How Two Organizations Are Bringing Hope and Care to Greece's Elderly," *The Huffington Post,* last modified January 10, 2017, accessed May 2017, www.huffingtonpost.com/entry/greece-elderly_us_561d6ed5e4b0c5a1ce60f1d2.

Levinson, D. R. "Adverse Events in Skilled Nursing Facilities: National Incidence Among Medicare Beneficiaries" Office of Inspector General, accessed September 2017, https://oig.hhs.gov/oei/reports/oei-06-11-00370.pdf.

Levy, M. "Audit Questions Enforcement of Nursing Home Staffing Levels," ABC 27 News, July 26, 2016, abc27.com/page/693/?cid=twitter_abc27News.

Lin, J. "Honor or Abandon: Societies' Treatment of Elderly Intrigues Scholar," UCLA Newsroom, January 7, 2010, accessed October 2016, http://newsroom.ucla.edu/stories/jared-diamond-on-aging-150571.

Liu, C. F., Subramanian, S., and Cromwell, J. "Impact of Global Bundled Payments on Hospital Costs of Coronary Artery Bypass Grafting," Journal of Health Care Finance 27, no. 4 (2001): 39–54, accessed March 2017, https://iths.pure.elsevier.com/.../impact-of-global-bundled-payments-on-hospital-costs-of-coronary-artery-bypass-grafting.

Long Term Care Community Coalition Memo: *Informed Consent for Psychotropic Medications:* "Bill to Ensure Informed Consent for The Use of Psychotropic Medication in Nursing Homes and Adult Care Facilities"_March 2017 accessed June 2017, http://www.nursinghome411.org/

"Long Term Care Facilities Assessment Instrument MDS 3.0 User's RAI Manual Version 1.13," Centers for Medicare & Medicaid Services, accessed February 2017, https://www. cms.gov/Medicare/Quality-Initiatives-Patient-Assessment-Instruments/NursingHomeQualityInits/Downloads/MDS-30-RAI-Manual-V113.pdf.

"Long-Term Care Facilities FAQs," Health Facilities Consumer Information System, accessed January 2017, http://hfcis.cd-Nph.ca.gov/faq/longtermcare.aspx.

Luczkiewocz MD, D. and Denall ANP, K. "Palliative Care…Goals of Care: DNR," Supportive Medical Partners Talk, accessed April 2017, http://www.chsbuffalo.org/files/pdf/Osteo%20 Lecture%20-%20Palliative%20Care%20DNR%20talk%20 5-2015.pdf.

Lundstrom, M., and Reese, P. "Unmasked: How California's Largest Nursing Home Chains Perform," *The Sacramento Bee*, November 8, 2014, accessed August 2016, http://media. sacbee.com/static/sinclair/Nursing1c/index.html.

Maguire, T. G., Newhouse, J. P., and Sinaiko, A.D. "An Economic History of Medicare Part C," *The Milbank Quarterly* 91, no. 1: 210, accessed April 2017 https://www.ncbi.nlm.nih.gov/ pubmed/21676024.

Malugani, M. "Battling Burnout in Nursing," Nursing Link, accessed March 2017, http://nursinglink.monster.com/benefits/articles/6239-battling-burnout-in-nursing.

"Man in Wheelchair, Left in the Sun at Florida Nursing Home, Dies," Fox News Health, accessed October 2016, http://www.foxnews.com/health/2016/05/03/man-in-wheelchair-left-in-sun-at-florida-nursing-home-dies.html.

"Mandatory Managed Care in New York May Lead to Poor Care in Nursing Homes," April 2014 Gallivan and Gallivan New York Nursing Home Abuse Lawyer blog, accessed May 2017, https://www.newyorknursinghomeabuselawyerblog.com/2014/04/report-mandatory-managed-care.html.

Martin, D. "Britain Should Be Ashamed of How It Treats Grandparents: Health Secretary Condemns Families' Neglect of Elderly," *The Daily Mail*, updated October 18, 2013, accessed November 2016, http://www.dailymail.co.uk/news/article-2465576/Health-Secretary-Jeremy-Hunt-condemns-elderly-neglect.html.

Martinez-Carter, K. "How the Elderly Are Treated around the World," *The Week*, July 2013, accessed September 2016, http://theweek.com/articles/462230/how-elderly-are-treated-around-world.

Mastrangelo, K. "Medicare Rehabilitation Medium and Low RUG Categories—Distinct Days," Harmony Healthcare, December 2013 accessed November 2016, http://www.harmony-health-care.com/blog/bid/100389/Medicare-Rehabilitation-Medium-and-Low-RUG-Categories-Distinct-Days.

McCoy, K. "Bank of America Fined $430M for Cash Misuse," *USA Today*, June 24, 2016.

"MDS RAI Version 3.0 Manual Chapter 3 Section G," Centers for Medicare & Medicaid Services, accessed January 2017, https://www.ahcancal.org/facility_operations/Documents/UpdatedFilesOct2010/Chapter%203%20-%20Section%20G%20V1.04%20Sept%202010.pdf.

Mechanic, R. E., and Altman, S. H. "Payment Reform Options: Episode Payment Is a Good Place to Start," *Health Affairs* 28, no. 2 (2009): 262–71, accessed May 2017, content.healthaffairs.org/content/28/2/w262.full.pdf+html.

"Medicaid Managed Care Enrollment Report," Medicaid.gov, accessed February 2017, https://www.medicaid.gov/medicaid/managed-care/enrollment/index.html.

"Medicare finalizes fiscal year 2018 payment & policy changes for skilled nursing facilities" July 2017 Centers for Medicare and Medicaid Services accessed October 2017, https://www.cms.gov/Newsroom/MediaReleaseDatabase/Fact-sheets/2017-Fact-Sheet-items/2017-07-31.html

"Medicare Fraud and Abuse: DOJ Continues to Promote Compliance with False Claims Act Guidance," US Government Accountability Office, accessed September 2017, www.gao.gov/new.items/d02546.pdf.

"*Medicare Payment Policy, Report to Congress,*" Section 2D March 2008 Medicare Payment Advisory Commission, accessed May 2017, www.medpac.gov/docs/default-source/reports/Mar08_EntireReport.pdf

"Medicare Reimbursement for Skilled Nursing Facilities Remains High for 2012 Despite Reductions in Overpayments," Center for Medicare Advocacy, accessed October 2016, http://www.medicareadvocacy.org/medicare-reimbursement-for-skilled-nursing-facilities-remains-high-for-2010-despite-reductions-in-overpayments/.

Meng, M., and Hunt, K. "New Chinese Law: Visit Your Parents," CNN, last modified July 2, 2013, accessed November 2016, www.cnn.com/2013/07/02/world/asia/china-elderly-law/index.html.

Mills, R. "Florida Moves to Close Second Facility Run by Owner of Nursing Home Where Eleven Died," *USA Today,* September 28, 2017, https://www.usatoday.com/story/news/nation-now/2017/09/28/florida-moves-close-second-facility-run-owner-nursing-home-where-11-died/715239001/.

Mollot, R. "Executive Summary: Safeguarding Residents and Program Integrity in NY State Nursing Homes," The Long-Term Care Community Coalition, last modified 2015, accessed September 2017, http://nursinghome411. org/?s=safeguarding.

Mollot, R. "Federal Requirements & Regulatory Provisions Relevant to Dementia Care & The Use of Antipsychotic Drugs" The Long Term Care Community Coalition 2013 accessed July 2017, http://www.susanwehrymd.com/uploads/5/8/3/4/5834405/antipsychotic_2013.pdf

Mollot, R., Butler, D., Baratt, V., Symkowski, J. "Informed Consent Rights in U.S. Nursing Homes: An Overview of State and Federal Requirements" The Long- Term Care Community Coalition September 2013 accessed April 2017 http://theconsumervoice.org/uploads/files/issues/ltccc-rpt-informed.pdf

Mollot, R., and Rudder, C. "Modifying the Case-Mix Medicaid Nursing Home System to Encourage Quality, Access and Efficiency" The Long Term Care Community Coalition Oct. 2009 accessed March 2017, http://theconsumervoice. org/uploads/files/events/Using-Medicaid-Reimbursement-System-Mollot-Rudder-PPT.pdf

Mollot, R. "The Long-Term Care Community Coalition," *The LTCCC Journal* 2, no. 4   (2016), 2–10, www.ltccc.org/news/.

Mongan, E. "Illinois Becomes the Fifth State to Allow Cameras in Nursing Home Rooms," *McKnights: The News You Need,* accessed August 2016, http://www.mcknights.com/news/ illinois-becomes-fifth-state-to-allow-cameras-in-nursing-home-rooms/article/434524/?webSyncID=2a2109e8-d644-2377-448a-0398bb1508d7&sessionGUID=2c8a31c4-ad18-09e7-58c5-12b202da724d.

"More on Productivity in Skilled Nursing Facilities," *The ASHA Leader* September 2014, Vol.19 accessed March 2017, leader. pubs.asha.org/article.aspx?articleid=901949.

Moss, F. E. *Too Old, Too Sick, Too Bad: Nursing Homes in America* (Germantown, MD: Aspen Publishing, 1977).

Mullman, R. "Sentosa Care's Expansion in NY," Abuse and Neglect, Advocacy, Staffing and Trial Themes, accessed October 2016, http://www.gpoliakoff.com/.

"National Partnership to Improve Dementia Care in Nursing Homes Centers on Medicare & Medicaid Services" Last modified 10/25/2017 accessed November 2017, https://www. cms.gov/Medicare/Provider-Enrollment-and-Certification/ SurveyCertificationGenInfo/National-Partnership-to-Improve_Dementia-Care-In-Nursing-Homes.html

National Consumer Voice for Quality Long-Term Care Revised Federal Nursing Home Regulations: Final Ruling accessed November 2017, http://theconsumervoice.org/issues/issue_details/proposed-revisions-to-the-federal-nursing-home-regulations.

"Nonfatal Occupational Injuries and Illnesses Requiring Days Away from Work, 2015," US Department of Labor Bureau of Labor Statistics, November 2016 accessed April 2017, https://www.bls.gov/news.release/osh2.nr0.htm.

"Non-Profit vs. For-Profit Nursing Homes: Is There a Difference in Care," Center for Medicare Advocacy, December 2011 accessed May 2017, http://www.medicareadvocacy.org/non-profit-vs-for-profit-nursing-homes-is-there-a-difference-in-care/.

"Nursing Home Administrator Education and Career Requirements," Study.com, accessed April 2017, http://study.com/nursing_home_administrator.html.

"Nursing Home Administrator Licensure Qualifications," New York State Department of Health, accessed March 2017, https://www.health.ny.gov/professionals/nursing_home_administrator/licensure_program/qualifications.htm.

Nursing Home Enforcement: Collection of Civil Monetary Penalties, Office of Inspector General, accessed August 2017, https://www.oig.hhs.gov/oei/reports/oei-06-03-00420.pdf.

"Nursing Home Operator to Pay $48 Million to Resolve Allegations that Six California Facilities billed for Unnecessary Therapy," US Department of Justice, accessed September 2017, https://www.justice.gov/opa/pr/nursing-home-operator-pay-48-million-resolve-allegations-six-california-facilities-billed.

"Nursing Home Residents at Risk," The Long-Term Care Community Coalition, accessed June 2017, http://www.ltccc.org.

"Nursing Homes Added to Federal Watch List for 'Grotesque' Abuse," Families for Better Care, accessed October 2016, http://familiesforbettercare.com/articles/nursing-homes-added-to-federal-watch-list-for-grotesque-abuse/.

"Nursing Homes Compete with Lavish Amenities for Short-Term Rehabilitation Residents," August 2015 Gallivan and Gallivan New York Nursing Home Abuse Lawyer Blog, accessed March 2017, https://www.newyorknursinghomeabuse-lawyerblog.com/2015/08/nursing-homes-compete-with-lav.html.

"Nursing Homes: Complexity of Private Investment Purchases Demonstrates Need for CMS to Improve the Usability and Completeness of Ownership Data," US Government Accountability Office, accessed August 2017, http://www.gao.gov/assets/320/310562.pdf.

"Nursing Homes, Private Investment Homes Sometimes Differ from Others in Deficiencies, Staffing, and Financial Performance," US Government Accountability Office, last modified July 2011, accessed May 2017, http://www.gao.gov/new.items/d11571.pdfancial.

Ochinko, W. "Nursing Home Quality: Findings from GAO Reports," National Health Policy Forum, accessed August 2017, http://www.nhpf.org/library/handouts/Ochinko.slides_03-25-10.pdf.

Ojo, O. "Problems with Use of a Foley Catheter in Enteral Tube Feeding," PubFacts, accessed May 2017, https://www.pub-facts.com/detail/24732987/Problems-with-use-of-a-Foley-catheter-in-enteral-tube-feeding.

O'Neill, J., and Rosen, A. L., *Professional Social Work Services in Skilled Nursing Facilities* (Washington, DC: National Association of Social Workers, 1998).

"Open-Ended Working Group on Ageing," United Nations Human Rights Office of the High Commissioner, accessed April 2017, https://social.un.org/ageing-working-group/.

"Oppose Efforts to Rollback and Delay the Nursing Home Rules" Sign a Letter to CMS! October 31, 2017 The National Consumer Voice for Quality Long-Term Care accessed November 2017, http://theconsumervoice.org/uploads/files/issues/CMS_letter_about_rollback_of_nursing_home_regulations_10-26-17.pdf

Pear, R. "Trump Moving to Impede Consumer Lawsuits Against Nursing Homes," *The New York Times*, August 19, 2017, accessed August 2017, https://www.nytimes.com/2017/08/18/us/politics/trump-impedes-consumer-lawsuits-against-nursing-homes-deregulation.html.

Pear, R. "Violations Reported at 94% of Nursing Homes," *New York Times*, September 29, 2008. accessed February 2017, www.nytimes.com/2008/09/30/us/30nursing.html

"Plan Benefits Comparison Chart—Comparing FIDA, PACE, MAP, and MLTC," New York State Department of Health, accessed December 2016, https://www.health.ny.gov/health_care/medicaid/redesign/fida/docs/plan_benefits_english.pdf.

"Poorly Performing Nursing Homes: Special Focus Facilities are Often Improving, but CMS's Program Could Be Strengthened," US Government Accountability Office, last modified April 19, 2010, accessed May 2017, http://www.gao.gov/products/GAO-10-197.

Pope, C. "Medicare's Single-Payer Experience," National Affairs, accessed August 2017, https://www.nationalaffairs.com/publications/detail/medicares-single-payer-experience.

Printup-Harms, C. "Aging Elders Among Native American Populations," Niagara County New York, accessed December 2016, http://www.niagaracounty.com/Portals/5/Images/June2010.pdf.

"Questionable Billing by Skilled Nursing Facilities," Office of Inspector General, OEI-02-09-00200 (Dec. 2010), accessed August 2017, http://oig.hhs.gov/oei/reports/oei-02-09-00202.pdf.

"Recovery Auditing in Medicare and Medicaid for Fiscal Year 2012," Centers for Medicare & Medicaid Services, accessed September 2017, https://www.cms.gov/Research-Statistics-Data-and-Systems/Monitoring-Programs/Medicare-FFS-Compliance-Programs/Recovery-Audit-Program/Downloads/Report-To-Congress-Recovery-Auditing-in-Medicare-and-Medicaid-for-Fiscal-Year-2012_013114.pdf.

"Resident Assessment Instrument Version 3.0 User's Manual," Centers for Medicare & Medicaid Services, accessed January 2017, https://www.cms.gov/Medicare/Quality-Initiatives-Patient-Assessment-Instruments/NursingHomeQuality-Inits/Downloads/MDS-30-RAI-Manual-V113.pdf.

Robinow, A. "The Potential of Global Payment: Insights from the Field," The Commonwealth Fund, accessed December 2016, http://www.commonwealthfund.org/~/media/Files/Publications/Fund%20Report/2010/Feb/1373_Robinow_potential_global_payment.pdf.

Rogers, S., and Komisar, H. *Who Needs Long-Term Care? Fact Sheet, Long-Term Care Financing Project* (Washington, DC: Georgetown University Press, 2003), http://www.aaltci.org/long-term-care-insurance/learning-center/long-term-care-statistics.php.

Runyeon, F. "As NY Shifts to For-Profit Nursing Homes, Abuse and Neglect Complaints Spike," New York Nonprofit Media, March 2016 accessed June 2016, http://nynmedia.com/news/as-ny-shifts-to-for-profit-nursing-homes-abuse-and-neglect-complaints-spike.

"Safe-Staffing Ratios: Benefiting Nurses and Patients," Department for Professional Employees, AFL-CIO Fact Sheet 2016 accessed June 2017, http://dpeaflcio.org/programs-publications/issue-fact-sheets/safe-staffing-ratios-benefiting-nurses-and-patients.

Satin, D. J., and Miles, J. "Performance-Based Bundled Payments: Potential Benefits and Burdens," *Minnesota Medicine* 92, no. 10 (2009)

Savitz, L. A., Jones, C. B., and Bernard, S. "Quality Indicators Sensitive to Nursing Staffing in Acute Care Settings," Advances in Patient Safety: From Research to Implementation, Vol. 4 2005 accessed January 2017, https://www.ncbi.nlm.nih.gov/books/NBK20600/.

"Seven Cultures that Celebrate Aging and Respect Their Elders," *The Huffington Post*, last modified May 16, 2015, accessed November 2016, https://www.huffingtonpost.com/2014/02/25/what-other-cultures-can-teach_n_4834228.html.

"Side-by-Side Comparison of Major Health Care Reform Proposals," Henry J. Kaiser Family Foundation, accessed April 2017, http://www.kff.org/health-reform/issue-brief/side-by-side-comparison-of-major-health-care-reform-proposals/.

"Skilled Nursing Facilities: Available Data Show Average Nursing Staff Time Changed Little after Medicare Payment Increase," US Government Accountability Office, accessed June 2017, http://www.gao.gov/new.items/d03176.pdf.

"Skilled Nursing Facility Price per Bed Soars to Record, Assisted Living Just Beats Last Year's Record," Irving Levin Associates Inc., accessed February 2017, https://products.levinassociates.com/aboutus/press-releases/pr1702scar22/.

"Skilled Nursing Facility (SNF) Prospective Payment System, PPS Legislative History," Centers for Medicare & Medicaid Services, Updated July 31, 2013, accessed November 2016, https://www.cms.gov/Medicare/Medicare-Fee-for-Service-Payment/SNFPPS/Downloads/Legislative_History_07302013.pdf.

"SNF Therapy Payment Models Base Year Final Summary," Centers for Medicare & Medicaid Services, accessed October 2016, https://www.cms.gov/Medicare/Medicare-Fee-for-Service-Payment/SNFPPS/Downloads/Summary_Report_20140501.pdf.

"Staffing Data Submission PBJ" Centers for Medicare & Medicaid Services Last modified 9/28/2017 accessed October 2017, https://www.cms.gov/Medicare/Quality-Initiatives-Patient-Assessment-Instruments/NursingHomeQualityInits/Staffing-Data-Submission-PBJ.html

"Statement on Post-Irma Nursing Home Deaths," The Long-Term Care Community Coalition, accessed October 2017, http://nursinghome411.org/statement-hurricane-irma/.

St. Hilaire, A. "Report Finds that Lack of Enforcement Allowed for Neglect at State Nursing Homes," ABC News, Pub. July 26, 2016 /Updated September 8, 2016, accessed November 2016, http://abc27.com/2016/07/26/report-finds-that-lack-of-enforcement-allowed-for-neglect-at-state-nursing-homes/.

"Sub-Acute and Long-Term Care Guide," IlluminAge Communication, accessed March 2017, http://www.illuminage.com/files/2014/05/Sub-Acute_CareGuide_Sample.pdf.

"Survey Protocol for Long Term Care Facilities—Part I," DOH survey Manual State Operations Manual Appendix P Rev 156, 6-10-16 Centers for Medicare & Medicaid Services, accessed November 2016, https://www.cms.gov/Regulations-and-Guidance/Guidance/Manuals/downloads/som107ap_p_ltcf.pdf.

"Technical Users' Guide for Nursing Home Compare Five-Star Quality Rating System" January 2017 accessed March 2017, https://www.cms.gov/Medicare/Provider-Enrollment-and-Certification/CertificationandComplianc/downloads/usersguide.pdf

"The Difference between Nursing Homes and Skilled Nursing Facilities," As You Age, accessed January 2017, http://www.asyouage.com/Difference_Between_Nursing_Homes_And_Skilled_Nursing_Facilities.html.

"The History of Nursing Homes: From Almshouses to Skilled Nursing," June 2015 Rincon del Rio: Abundant Living Successful Aging, accessed August 2016, http://rincondelrio.com/info-for-seniors/the-history-of-nursing-homes-from-almshouses-to-skilled-nursing/.

"The Spirit of America," American Health Care Association, accessed July 2017, https://www.ahcancal.org/events/national_nursing_home_week/.

Thomas, K. "In Race for Medicare Dollars, Nursing Home Care May Lag," *New York Times*, April 14, 2015, accessed June 2017, https://www.nytimes.com/2015/04/15/business/as-nursing-homes-chase-lucrative-patients-quality-of-care-is-said-to-lag.html.

Thomas, K. "Medicare Star Ratings Allow Nursing Homes to Game the System," *New York Times*, August 24, 2014. accessed June 2017, https://www.nytimes.com/2014/.../medicare-star-ratings-allow-nursing-homes-to-game-the-system

Thomas, W. C. *Nursing Homes and Public Policy* (Ithaca, NY: Cornell University Press, 1969)

"Transitions to Care," Care Conversations, accessed June 2017, https://careconversations.org/transition-care.

Tullis, R. L. *Benjamin Nathan Cardoza: Jurist, Philosopher, Humanitarian* Louisiana Law Review (1938) Volume 1/Number1 accessed September 2017, http://digitalcommons.law.lsu.edu/lalrev/vol1/iss1/19

Turnbaum, H. "Federal Nursing Home Reform Act from the Omnibus Budget Reconciliation Act of 1987 or OBRA '87 Summary 2016," NC Department of Health and Human Services, accessed September 2016, http://www.ncmust.com/doclib/OBRA87summary.pdf.

"Update of State Operations Manual (SOM) Chapter 5, Complaint Investigation," Centers for Medicare & Medicaid Services, last modified April 19, 2013, accessed March 2017, https://www.cms.gov/Medicare/Provider-Enrollment-and-Certification/SurveyCertificationGenInfo/Downloads/Survey-and-Cert-Letter-13-27.pdf.

"US Census Bureau Statistical Abstract of the United States: 2000," US Census Bureau, accessed September 2017, http://www.census.gov/prod/2004pubs/.

"US Nursing Assistants Employed in Nursing Homes: Key Facts," PHI, accessed September 2016, https://phinational.org/sites/default/files/phi-nursing-assistants-key-facts.pdf.

Virtanen, M., Ferrie, J., Singh-Manoux, A., Shipley, M., Vahtera, J., Marmot, M., and Kivimäki, M. "Overtime Work and Incident Coronary Heart Disease: The Whitehall II Prospective Cohort Study," *European Heart Journal* 31, no. 14 (2010): 1737–44, accessed June 2017, http://www.hal.inserm.fr/inserm-00488827.

Ward, B. "Third Generation Country, A Practical Guide to Raising Children with Great Values," accessed January 2017, https://www.values.com/inspirational-quotes/3002-we-were-taught-to-respect-elders-.

Ward PhD, R. S. "RE: Challenges Facing Physical Therapists in the Skilled Nursing Facility Setting," American Physical Therapy Association, accessed March 2017, https://www.apta.org/uploadedFiles/APTAorg/Payment/Medicare/Coding_and_Billing/SNF/Comments/APTAComments_SNF_072811.pdf.

Watson, S.T., "Below-Average Staffing Hurt the Overall Ratings at Some Area Nursing Homes," *The Buffalo News,* HighBeam Research August 21, 2016, accessed April 2017, https://www.highbeam.com/publications/the-buffalo-news-buffalo-ny.../aug-21-2016

Wells, J., and Harrington, C. "Information on Affordable Care Act Provisions to Improve Nursing Home Transparency, Care Quality, and Abuse Prevention," Kaiser Commission on Medicaid and the Uninsured, accessed June 2017, https://kaiserfamilyfoundation.files.wordpress.com/2013/02/8406.pdf.

"When Short-Term Rehab Turns into a Long-Term Stay," Next Step in Care: Family, Caregivers, & Health Care Professionals Working Together, accessed April 2017, https://www.nextstepincare.org/uploads/File/Guides/Rehabilitation/ST_to_LT/Rehab_To_Long_Term_Stay.pdf.

White Feather "Native American Beliefs," *Inter-Tribal Times*, last modified October 1994, accessed December 2016, http://www.home.earthlink.net/~tessia/Native.html.

White, J. "New York Case Mix," PostAcute Consulting, accessed January 2017, http://nyshfa.org/files/2013/07/PowerPointHandout.pdf.

Wikipedia, s.v. "Bundled Payment," accessed February 2017, https://en.wikipedia.org/wiki/Bundled_payment.

Wikipedia, s.v. "Medicare (United States)," accessed September 2017, https://en.wikipedia.org/wiki/Medicare_(United_States).

Wikipedia, s.v. "Old Age," accessed October 2016, https://en.wikipedia.org/wiki/Old_age.

Weixel, N. *"Lawmakers Unveil Draft Legislation to Reform Post-Acute Care Payments"* Bloomberg BNA March 19, 2014 accessed October 2017, https://www.bna.com/lawmakers-unveil-draft-n17179885866/

Wilcsher, K. "French Tighten Law to Ensure Families Keep Eye on Elderly Parents" Feb 18, 2004 accessed Oct 2016, http://www.theage.com.au/articles/2004/02/15/1076779835689.html

Wilsher, K. "French Forced to Care for Elderly Parents," Fairfax Digital, last modified February 16, 2004, accessed October 2016, http://www.theage.com.au/articles/ 2004/02/15/1076779835689.html.

Wright, O. "'Our National Shame': Health Secretary Jeremy Hunt Blasts British Society's Neglect of Its Elderly," *Independent*, last modified October 17, 2013, accessed October 2016, http:// www.independent.co.uk/news/uk/politics/our-national- shame-health-secretary-jeremy-hunt-blasts-british-society-s- neglect-of-its-elderly-8887532.html.

Zhang, N. J., L. Unruh, R. Liu, and T. T. Wan. "Minimum Nurse Staffing Ratios for Nursing Homes," *Nurse Economics* 2006 March-April; 24, no. 2: 78–85, accessed September 2017, https://www.ncbi.nlm.nih.gov/pubmed/16676750.